Aging Well

A Reality Now Possible Through

Intermittent Fasting and Proper Eating

By Dr. Grady L Goolsby

First Printing, 2019

Grady L Goolsby LLC
Rockledge, FL 32955

This book is not intended or implied to be a substitute for professional medical advice of physicians. The information included is for general or educational purposes only. The reader should consult their physician in matters relating to his/her health and particularly with respect to this information or any other symptoms that may require diagnosis or medical attention. Reading the information in this book does not create a physician-patient relationship.

Contents

Acknowledgements

To Rochelle, my wife, and all my family members who have inspired and encouraged me in this endeavor.

Special thanks to Robb Hawks, my brother-in-law (the Bob guy) whose expertise is unsurpassed when it comes to writing and publishing.

A Note from the Author.

It has now been over 41 years that I have been in the practice of functional and nutritional medicine. Through these years I have extensively studied and researched all kinds of therapies, modalities, diets, and remedies; some good and some not so good. We are constantly bludgeoned with the next "greatest" pill, potion, diet plan, miracle nutrient, or exercise program. So, as you can imagine, I'm not easily impressed with new ideas and therapies, especially at this point in my career. Therefore, the concept of any kind of fasting was never utilized nor recommended to my patients because my personal experiences with fasting were not always good. **That has changed.**

There is now a plethora of well-researched information on diet, health and fasting that is making monumental headway in the treatment of many health conditions, including some major breakthroughs in obesity, type 2 diabetes, cardiovascular disease, high blood pressure and aging. This got my attention! As I began to dig into this new emerging research, I was amazed. I was shocked that this information was not more widely known. It's almost like they were trying to hide this information from us. I can now honestly say that I am impressed. And as a result, I have become passionate about gathering information on "intermittent fasting" for the purpose of designing a concise format of implementation for my patients and to anyone else that is interested. This has also led me to a wake-up call of my own. Consider this.

My wife and I, as we enter our mid-60's, realize we are on a journey to our 70's, 80's and beyond. The question is what kind of health are we going to be in when we get there. I believe you will see in this book that there is now a viable way that empowers you to take control of your health, backed up by good research thereby giving you a great chance to "Age Well". Come join us in this journey.

Dr. Grady L Goolsby
July 1, 2019

Preface

This is a book of implementation. I constantly have patients query me concerning diets, foods and fasting. There is a multitude of diet and food information in books as well as online which unfortunately has led to a lot of confusion. What should I do, when should I do it; Paleo, Keto, Atkins, no carb, low carb, high fat, low fat, no fat, and on and on it goes? My clinical experience confirms that this confusion has led to low compliance and follow through, ultimately leading to failure and then on to bad health.

In this book I will first give a synopsis of the current peer reviewed research on diet, Intermittent Fasting and hormonal (mainly Insulin) influence as it relates to our health. Then I will present to you a clear and concise method of implementation in order to hopefully dispel the confusion that is apparent. *For those of you that are ready to jump right in and get started, go to chapter 13. This is a brief review of the book and Quick Start Chapter.* Then I would encourage you to read the book from the beginning.

As you start this journey, I want to encourage you to *keep your eye on the ball.* And what I mean by that is even though you can expect weight loss, lower blood sugar, decrease inflammation, lower blood pressure and more; these are really just the nice side effects of the process. The goal, *or the ball,* is the pursuit of good health through Intermittent Fasting and the eating of good whole foods that will allow you to "Age Well". The weight loss and all of the other health benefits will then become the fruit of the process. This will keep you encouraged and engaged on those days that progress seems slow or the weight or sugar or other problems are not moving as fast as you would like. Remember, Intermittent Fasting literally allows the body to reboot itself back to its original design and function. This is really what we are after. And it takes time. So, hang in there. You got this. I know you can do it.

CHAPTER 1 "Bob and the Doc"

'BOB"

Everyone has their own opinion as to what "living well" is. My brother-in-law, let's call him Bob, has "lived well" his entire life. He didn't start out obese. Most people do not. It sort of crept up on him. He was athletic in high school and could eat whatever he wanted, and as much as he wanted, and never gained a pound. But eventually he got his first desk job and gained 10 pounds that first year. Next came love, and then came marriage, and with the marriage he picked up another 15 pounds the first year. Forty years later and Bob is not just overweight, he is obese. His living well has set him up not to age well.

Now Bob is a little OCD, that is, obsessive compulsive. Where most thin people can stop eating when they are full, Bob struggles with obsessing over the foods he loves the most. Bob doesn't think twice about vegetables, but put a steaming pizza on the table and Bob is a goner. He loads a couple of slices onto a plate, shoves the pizza box into the refrigerator, and then grabbing up a soft drink, he heads to the family room to eat his dinner and binge watch some TV. Soon Bob is washing down the last bite of pizza with the last of his soda. All is good . . . until the show ends. In the silence as the next episode is loading, Bob hears a small voice coming from the kitchen. At first it is just a whisper at the back of his mind. But it grows louder and louder. "Eat me!" Bob tries to ignore it, but it won't go away. "Eat me!" The pizza in the refrigerator is calling to him and getting stronger and more demanding. Fiddling with the TV remote control does not make the voice go away. If only the next episode would load faster. But it is not to be. Bob is obsessing over the pizza laying just 25 feet away. It's calling out to him. The obsession has now become a compulsion. Jumping out of his chair he quickly reloads his plate with two more slices of pizza and tops off his glass with another can of soda. This sequence will be repeated until the entire pizza has been devoured. While Bob sits and enjoys the last bite of the last piece of pizza, he is completely unaware of the chaos that is going on deep in his burgeoning belly. You see, Bob's body is a complete microcosm designed to operate as a complex and balanced machine. The pizza and soda have dumped into his stomach where the digestive process have broken everything down into manageable raw materials for his body's power plant. The pizza and soda are quickly converted to sugar. Then a large conveyor belt hauls the sugar up out of the intestines and into the power plant, his liver. This is where the chaos is happening. The refined flour used to make the pizza dough converted almost instantly to sugar. The sugar in the soft drink didn't even require conversion. The conveyor belt is having to operate at full speed to keep up with the processing down in the intestines. As the sugar begins to pile up, an alarm sounds as the liver foreman sends a text to the pancreas. "Send help! We're being overrun!" Meanwhile, there is a bunch of tired and exhausted little guys in gray suits and yellow hardhats still on the job. The large "I" on their gray uniforms shows that they are part of the insulin crew. They are exhausted. They just wrapped up their first shift processing Bob's first two pieces of pizza. Now the alarm has been sounded, another crew of the "I" brigade, grab up their shovels and a fresh box of trash bags, and rush to the liver. Arriving at the liver they immediately recognize the problem. The conveyor belt is out of control and spraying sugar all over the liver. Some of the "I" guys shovel a portion of the sugar into storage bins in the liver. The rest of the "I" guys starts shoveling sugar out into the nearest artery. But the arteries are designed to only operate with so much sugar. But the crew is exhausted. They are making mistakes. Everyone is shoveling as fast as they can and they are still falling behind. No one notices that the sugar level in the blood is exceeding manufacturer's specification. At these levels Bob is unknowingly becoming diabetic. Finally, the crew realizes they have overstocked the blood system. They are going to have to do something else with all of this sugar. One guy rolls out a conversion machine. He gives the starter cable a couple of pulls and it quickly comes to life. The crew recognizes the sound and divides up into two teams. The first team shovels the sugar into the converter as fast as they can. Fat comes shooting out of the other side of the converter. The other half of the crew shovels the fat as fast as they can into huge piles. But the liver is running out of storage space. There is only one thing left to do. They pull out their boxes of trash bags and begin to shovel the fat into the bags. Before long the bags are piling up. The liver is in trouble. "Alright guys, let's start sending this excess to the landfill." The foreman orders. The crew lines up in a bucket brigade sticking storage labels on the bags and then dumping them into the blood system. The bags of fat float along until they reach the landfill where another crew pulls them out of the blood stream and stashes them away. "Gee, you would think the "I" Crew had sent enough of this stuff," one of the landfill workers complains. "Shut up and throw it on the pile," his partner responds. And the landfill, that is Bob's belly, just gets bigger and bigger and bigger.

And that is exactly what is happening.

Well, sort of.

"The DOC"

Bob is in trouble. All of his life choices are setting him up NOT to "age well." Although he has tried various diets over the years none of them has addressed the insulin problem.

INSULIN, yes this is the hormone that everyone refers to when discussing diabetes. It's the hormone that's produced in the pancreas and is generally known as a balancer of blood sugar levels. But very few people understand the significance of insulin levels in general health as it pertains to such maladies as obesity, type 2 diabetes, high blood pressure and cardiovascular disease to name just a few. This is the factor that has been missing from all of the diets, diet plans, weight loss plans, diabetic food plans and any other plan that concerns health, longevity, or aging. Or, at least it has been under emphasized.

Most doctors must be voracious readers to stay current in their practices. Bob has just rolled his eyes when I mentioned the latest conference I attended or thousand-page study I had digested. There is enormous research in the study of insulin. But no one study puts it all together. Then it happened. I discovered research which revealed how obesity, as well as many other health problems, were simply being caused by too much insulin in the blood, which is a condition called hyperinsulinemia. Other research on the reversal of type 2 diabetes was absolutely stunning. [1] We have known, for quite some time, about hyperinsulinemia and the problems that it causes, however, there has been some disagreement on the mechanism in which it creates disease. Several studies have now proven that hyperinsulinemia, and the cascade of events that occur concurrently, is a huge trigger of the above-mentioned diseases. [2] This triggered a giant "Wow Moment" in my thinking. I said to myself, "Can it be this simple? How did we not understand this before now?

So, I'm just going to say it right off the bat; if your pursuit of health and aging well, does not include dealing with insulin levels in the body, your success is going to be temporary at best; and a total failure at worse. Insulin levels have to be considered whether you are trying to lose weight, reverse type II diabetes or improve cardiovascular health. Arthritis, chronic fatigue syndrome, autoimmune problems, polycystic ovary syndrome and just about any of the other chronic conditions of the day, appear to have an insulin connection as well.

You see, insulin is actually the controlling factor of where fat and sugar end up in the body and whether it's being stored or burned. You can look at it as a gatekeeper. Think of it this way:

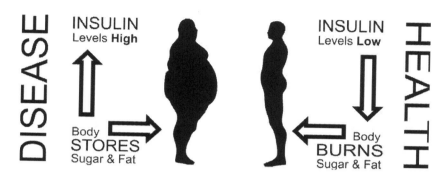

Bob has an insulin problem. He has become hyperinsulinemic. His pancreas is exhausted. Rather than metering out the proportional amount of insulin needed to control his blood sugar, the pancreas in a continual panic mode, dumps excessive insulin in the body to deal with excess sugar. He has tried many different diet plans, most of which were successful in the short run, but fail in the long run, because the hormonal factor, primarily insulin, is never addressed. Even though Bob lowered calories, carbs and so on; nothing was ever done to address the hyperinsulinemia. Bob actually has lost a lot of weight over the years. But he was never able to sustain the "new him". Since he never addressed the insulin issue, Bob slowly regained the weight he lost, plus a few additional pounds for good measure. Sound familiar? This is the infamous yo-yo dieting.

So, if insulin levels are the problem, how do we control them? How do we reset the body and lower insulin? The answer is to <u>not</u> eat. We call this fasting; that means going without food for a period of time. That lowers the insulin levels and begins to allow the body to reset which gives the pancreas and liver a break. These vital organs need a chance to rest-up and reset. Studies have shown that regular fasting is the key to this desired reset. This is what is called, "intermittent fasting."

Intermittent fasting has been around for quite some time. However, recent, newly discovered research, has shed new light on how and why it works so well. We knew it had some benefit but we didn't always know the mechanics behind the results. Also, there was a lot of confusion on the methods of implementation such as the amount of time of the fast, and the intervals between fasting and eating. There is now enough data and experience to help us navigate these variables. So, by increasing the time intervals between eating meals, we decrease the levels of insulin in the blood. This is key. As a result, we see amazing physiological changes occurring for the better.

Intermittent fasting creates <u>greater insulin sensitivity</u> which allows the body to regain better function.[3] Greater insulin sensitivity means it takes less insulin to control the sugar levels in the body. This is **huge**. Medicine and all healthcare providers have longed to accomplish this, but to no avail, until now.

At the root of Bob's problems is "insulin resistance". This is the opposite of insulin sensitivity. Insulin resistance keeps sugar levels high and makes them difficult to control. Poor Bob, the "I Guys" in his liver were shoveling sugar into his bloodstream. Soon all of the cells in the body have reached sugar saturation. Can you imagine one of the "I Guys" setting up a lemonade delivery truck going up and down Bob's arteries? In the back of the truck there is a massive pile of sugar. There's a sign on the side of the truck which reads, "Get Your Free Sugar Here." As well as blasting it out on a loudspeaker. But as the truck rolls by, the cells call out to him saying that they are full. They had loaded up on sugar, to the point of overload, on previous deliveries. Eventually the pile of sugar in the back of the lemonade truck is just dumped in the bloodstream.

And there you go, Bob has just experienced Insulin resistance. <u>Insulin resistance</u> means that insulin has lost its ability to push any more sugar into the cells of the body because the cells are completely full and overloaded. Now the excess sugar spills over into the bloodstream causing high sugar levels. Intermittent fasting allows the excess sugar to burn off. As the sugar burns off, the insulin resistance will decrease, and the body will return back to greater insulin sensitivity. You see, if you can control insulin resistance you can control sugar, and if you can control sugar, you can control fat production. It's that simple. Regaining sensitivity to insulin, enables the body to burn excess sugar and fat, leading to weight loss and lower sugar levels. So far, no medications have been able to accomplish this in and by themselves. Intermittent fasting and eating whole foods is simply unsurpassed in being able to reach these goals.

I practice intermittent fasting. No, I'm not the fat guy on the cover. I am the ideal weight for my body type and height. By all standards, I am healthy. Why should someone like me practice intermittent fasting? The answer is simple. I want to age well. Doing an 18 - 24 hour fast once or twice a week, is good for the purpose of resetting the mitochondria found in all of our cells. The mitochondria are the energy makers of each cell in our body. They produce all of the energy that keeps the cell operating. Without them, the cell will die. I don't want to get too technical, but there is a lot of metabolic activity that occurs in the mitochondria and more and more doctors and researchers agree that if you can keep the mitochondria healthy, then you will have a much better chance at recapturing and maintaining your health. When mitochondria get corrupted; whether it's by viruses, bacteria, toxic insult, heavy metals, or hormonal insult, including high insulin levels; it begins to create an inflammatory response which ultimately leads to disease. So, protecting the mitochondria becomes paramount whether you're overweight or thin. Intermittent fasting accomplishes this by detoxing the cells and resetting mitochondrial function thereby allowing them to recover. It also empties the cells of the excess sugars and fats that have accumulated from high insulin levels. I believe this is the key to maintaining good health and longevity.

Intermittent fasting literally allows the body to reboot itself back to its original design and function.

Do you want to age well? Perhaps adding decades to your life while first improving and then maintaining your health? The following chapters will walk you through the concepts, methods, and typical practices necessary for you to "age well."

(1) E. L. Lim, K. G. Hollingsworth, B. S. Aribisala, M. J. Chen, J. C. Mathers, and R. Taylor.
"Reversal of type 2 diabetes: normalization of beta cell function in association with decreased pancreas and liver triacylglycerol."
Diabetologia. 2011 Oct; 54(10):2506–2514

(2) Jennifer M. Perkins, Nino G. Joy, Donna B. Tate, and Stephen N. Davis.
"Acute effects of hyperinsulinemia and hyperglycemia on vascular inflammatory biomarkers and endothelial function in overweight and obese humans."
Am J Physiol Endocrinol Metab. 2015 Jul 15; 309(2): E168–E176.

(3) Elizabeth F.Sutton, Robbie Beyl Kate S.Early William T.Cefalu1 EricRavussin Courtney M.Peterson.
"Early Time-Restricted Feeding Improves Insulin Sensitivity, Blood Pressure, Oxidative Stress Even without Weight Loss in Men with Prediabetes."
Cell Metabolism. Volume 27, Issue 6, 5 June 2018, Pages 1212-1221.e3

CHAPTER 2 "Sugar"

Great news! Bob has finally decided to do something about his blood sugar. Eating healthy will be his first step. No more of those evil sugar loaded soft drinks for him. No sir-ree bob. Nope. He is going nat-ur-al. The next morning its up bright and early. A bowl of Honey Oats cereal washed down with a big glass of orange juice. Oats and OJ. Now that is healthy! And at lunch? No more white bread for Bob. It's peanut butter and jelly (jelly is fruit, right?) on whole wheat bread. Again, Bob has given up soft drinks and so he washes the PB&J down with a 16oz bottle of "natural" apple juice. Bob just knows that this new healthy food lifestyle will have him fixed up in no time at all. Right? Uh, sorry Bob. Wrong!

Sugar, Sugar, Sugar; everybody's talking about it. Everybody knows it's bad but unfortunately it still remains a huge part of our diets. There is sugar in almost everything we eat. Some of the sugar is natural to the food. In other products sugar has been added. It is a given: excess sugar is fattening. Most people would also agree that sugar is at the root of many of our ailments and health conditions. Remember Bob's story? Sugar, and the resulting insulin resistance, is the main culprit in his overweight and unhealthy condition.

There are **two** main sugars that are predominant in our bodies.

Glucose

Glucose is the main sugar found in the blood that circulates throughout the body. It is the main source of energy for the brain, muscle, and blood cells. As well as circulating in the blood, glucose can also be stored in the liver in the form of glycogen. Dr. Robert Lustig M.D., a pediatric endocrinologist, calls glucose *the energy of life.*[1] The liver can also produce its own glucose by a process called gluconeogenesis (which means making new glucose). When the blood levels of glucose begin to get too low the liver will then convert glycogen into glucose to bring blood levels back to normal range.

Fructose

Fructose is a sugar that's naturally found in fruit. It can only be metabolized in the liver and does not circulate in the blood. The tissues of the body, particularly the brain and muscles, cannot use fructose for energy. Fructose does not affect the glucose levels of the blood either which makes it appealing to the diabetic diet. This is a big mistake as we will see shortly. Bob assumed that since fructose doesn't affect blood glucose levels, it must be something safe to consume. But there is a nasty downside to fructose.

When glucose and fructose are combined it's called **sucrose** which is commonly known as table sugar. Sucrose is composed of 50 percent glucose and 50 percent fructose. Carbohydrates are sugars that are chained together. High- fructose corn syrup is 55 percent fructose and 45 percent glucose.

Bob is in trouble. He has been drinking orange and apple juice like it is water. That 16 oz apple juice contains over 63 grams of sugar, and the orange juice is not much better containing almost 52 grams of sugar. 50 percent of the sugar in orange juice is glucose, and 50 percent is fructose. Consuming large amounts is problematic in our diet, especially if your trying to lose weight. But fructose has a dark side as many researchers now refer to fructose as a poison.

How can that be when we've heard all of our lives that fruits and vegetables should be one of the main staples of our diet, especially in the realm of natural healthy eating. The answer is in the way fructose is processed in the liver. Dr. Robert Lustig's 2009 speech *The Bitter Truth* exposed the truth about fructose and how it is metabolized in the liver and why it becomes toxic. [1] Fructose can only be metabolized in the liver.

When fructose enters the liver, it gets changed into fat, and this fat, in high enough levels, will begin to develop a fatty liver. Fructose has been stated in many publications to be five to ten times more likely to cause a fatty liver. [2] This fatty liver will then develop into and cause insulin resistance in the liver. Remember, insulin resistance is the condition where there is no more room in the cells of the body for sugar. They are full. Not another molecule can be jammed in. This insulin resistance causes the pancreas to produce even more insulin leading to even higher insulin levels. Continued high insulin levels attempt to store more sugar and fat in the liver and the cells of the body causing even more insulin resistance leading to even higher insulin levels and around and around we go. It gets totally out of control. Hello type 2 diabetes. This damages the liver in a way similar to the effects of alcohol which is a well-known toxin to the liver. [1] The liver then has to get rid of this excess fat mainly by sending it out into our fat cells which causes us to gain weight. So, as we can see this creates another impediment in our quest for lowering insulin levels in the blood. Remember, it's the insulin levels in the bloodstream that must be lowered in order to allow us to lose weight and control our diabetic situations.

Uh oh. It sounds like Bob's new diet is not quite as healthy as he thought. Can it possibly get worse? It has also been shown that fructose creates oxidative damage to our cells. This creates inflammation which can lead to a plethora of chronic degenerative diseases associated with the metabolic syndrome (obesity, diabetes, heart disease) as well as arthritis, inflammatory bowel disease, and small intestinal bacterial overgrowth. The ensuing liver damage, caused by fructose, can also cause a condition called dyslipidemia, which causes your blood lipid levels (cholesterol, triglycerides) to increase as well as causing an increase in liver enzymes in your blood lab results. This indicates that your liver is now in serious trouble with the possibility of being diseased.

The processing of fructose, in the liver, also blocks the production of nitric oxide (NO) in the blood vessels. This is highly significant because nitric oxide is the substance, in the lining of the blood vessels, that relaxes the blood vessels themselves. This keeps your blood pressure down. So, if fructose is blocking the production of nitric oxide, you end up with hypertension (high blood pressure). [1,5] Since we have a hypertension epidemic in this country, it might be a good idea to lay off the sugars especially fructose. While on the subject of blood pressure, studies have also shown that hyperinsulinemia also causes blood vessels to constrict resulting in increased blood pressure. [3]

Excess fructose affects brain functioning, especially as it relates to appetite regulation and function. This occurs as a result of **leptin**, which is a hormone that controls appetite, which signals the body and tells it that it has had enough to eat. So, fructose causes the brain to not get the signal, therefore you never feel full when eating foods containing fructose which leads to overeating and weight gain. [4]

While short-term consumption of fructose doesn't seem to be a problem, it's the cumulative effects over months and years that begin to add up causing a lot of the above-mentioned problems. This is the flaw in many of the studies on fructose which show short-term consumption of fructose causes no apparent problems mainly because it doesn't raise the levels of glucose in the blood and is not high on the glycemic index. Therefore, the negative effects of fructose are completely hidden.

SO, WHAT DO WE DO?
Does this mean we should never eat fruit again? Well, it depends. If you want to lose weight or are trying not to gain weight, you should remove all sugars from your diet. If you have any kind of active

disease or autoimmune condition, you should not consume sugar of any kind. If you like your weight level, small amounts of fruit would be permissible but only in the full fruit form not in the form of juices. Fruit juices are way too high in fructose and have no fiber. Fiber is the antidote to the toxin of fructose and helps to offset some of the harmful effects. Stay away from any drinks that contain high fructose corn syrup. Statistics are showing that this is a major cause of the obesity epidemic in this country, particularly in children. Artificial sweeteners are equally bad. Although they do not result in immediate insulin rise, they contribute to a variety of issues that can cause health problems. Reduce your artificial sweetener intake to a minimum. Eventually you might discover you just don't need it.   Watch out for what goes into various smoothie type drinks that many consume for breakfast and sometimes use for full meal replacement. The levels of hidden fructose can be significant.

Aging well is going to require that we eliminate or greatly reduce sugar from our diet.

(1) Lustig,R. Sugar: "the bitter truth." You Tube. Available from: https://www.youtube.com/watch?v=dBnniua6-oM Accessed 2019, May 18.

(2) Faeh D, et al.
"Effect of fructose Overfeeding and Fish Oil Administration on Hepatic De Novo Lipogenesis and Insulin Sensitivity in Healthy Men",
Diabetes 2005 Jul; 54(7): 1907-1913.

(3) Bönner G,
"Hyperinsulinemia, insulin resistance, and hypertension."
J Cardiovasc Pharmacol. 1994;24 Suppl 2:S39-49.

(4) Katrien Lowette, Lina Roosen, Jan Tack, and Pieter Vanden Berghe.
"Effects of High-Fructos Diets on Central Appetite Signaling and Cognitive Function."
Front Nutr. 2015; 2: 5.

(5) Alice Victoria Klein and Hosen Kiat. "The mechanisms underlying fructose-induced hypertension: a review".
J Hypertens. 2015 May; 33(5): 912–920.

CHAPTER 3 "The Benefits of Fasting"

Just what are the benefits of fasting? The most obvious benefit is that carbohydrate intake is decreased. Carbohydrates are a number of chemical compounds found in foods that are sugar, starch, and cellulose. Most carbohydrates can be broken down in the digestive process and turned into sugars. Thus, fasting reduces carbohydrate intake which results in less sugar in the body which lowers insulin and results in weight loss. It makes sense that if we restrict the intake of food, particularly sugars and carbohydrates, we're going to begin to lose weight.

Other benefits were seen in a 2018 study involving mice. One group of mice were allowed to eat as much as they wanted whenever they wanted. The second group of mice were only allowed to eat once every 24 hours. The mice that were fasted 24 hours and fed only once per day, showed improvement in overall health. They also experienced delays in age related damage to the liver and other organs. The study goes on to say that glucose and insulin levels showed significant improvement "Increasing daily fasting times, without a reduction of calories and regardless of the type of diet consumed, resulted in overall improvements in health and survival in male mice," said Rafael de Cabo, the study's leader.

"Perhaps this extended daily fasting period enables repair and maintenance mechanisms that would be absent in a continuous exposure to food." [6]

Similar results have been shown in people who practice intermittent fasting such as:

1. Increases fat burning
2. Induced weight loss
3. Lowered blood sugar levels
4. Improved insulin sensitivity [1]
5. Lowers blood fats including cholesterol and triglycerides

There are additional long-term benefits that are key factors in "aging well".

- Decreases inflammation
- Allows the body to shift into a healing mode
- Slows down our aging process thus increases our longevity [2]
- Seems to improve dementia and Alzheimer's disease

One of the surprising results of intermittent fasting is an increase in energy. Anne is one of my patients. Her health had slowly deteriorated to such a point that at the age of 36 she had reached a level of chronic fatigue that was becoming debilitating. She would wake each morning tired, work through the morning tired, and by 3 in the afternoon fall into her bed exhausted. Waking in the early evening she would eat a meal and soon be back in bed facing the same routine the next day. Her body was a mess swelling with the retention of fluids and constantly fighting inflammation demonstrated by the low-grade fevers she would run 4-7 days a week. Regular blood tests revealed nothing. A more detailed blood test eventually revealed 23 separate issues. We put Anne on a specific eating plan coupled with intermittent fasting augmented with specific nutritional supplements. The swelling and inflammation rapidly disappeared. Her energy level not only returned to normal, but she now is up and about all day and going on walks with her husband almost every day. Anne experienced a total turn around plus an energy increase.

It has been my personal experience that the initial result of intermittent fasting is improved mental & spiritual clarity. Now, I am the skinny guy. Why am I fasting? It's simple. I want to age well. But I also physically feel better with increased energy. Who wouldn't want increased clarity and energy? My wife and I are not alone in this experience. My patients have reported these same improvements in their own lives as they establish the regimen of intermittent fasting.

Now, back to Bob. Bob desperately needs to lose weight. The truth is the majority of those who live in western civilization need to lose weight. But he doesn't "feel good." He doesn't seem to have the energy or focus needed to succeed in an eating lifestyle change. Bob feels lousy and so he eats. But instead of feeling better, his energy levels drop and instead of "getting up and going," he ends up sitting down and "vegging." For Bob the obvious solution is to begin intermittent fasting. He would then be positioned to see a rise in energy and mental focus. The fasting also sets up his body for protracted weight loss. All of these immediate improvements are tied to burning off excess glucose and reducing insulin. Bob has taken the first step towards aging well. If we can keep him on target his aging process will slow down which increases his longevity. All of these benefits of intermittent fasting result from decreased inflammation in the body; improvements in the cholesterol and triglycerides levels while cleansing the body of toxins, and generally de-stressing the functions of the body.

Bob has allowed his body to get into a sorry state of being. He needs to do something immediately.

Instead of his body functioning as God designed it, it is in chaos. His many specialist doctors have prescribed numerous medications to treat sugar levels, high cholesterol, and high blood pressure. They really haven't made a difference. Bob needs to get his body out of the chaos and into a healthy metabolic mode where it's no longer reacting to the chaos. Now his body can more efficiently fight off disease processes. If he cannot change the state of his metabolic chaos, he will open himself up to many of the modern diseases of western civilization such as cardiovascular disease, high blood pressure, type 2 diabetes, Alzheimer's disease, dementia and arthritis. Bob needs to begin intermittent fasting at once. Bob needs to allow his body to "reboot" itself back to its original design and function.

Perhaps one of the biggest benefits of intermittent fasting is financial. Bob's pantry is full of various diet food program products. There are shake mixes, snack bars, food additives, and boxes of "fast start" diet products from about every popular "lose weight fast" system on the internet. Yup, Bob and his family have spent a small fortune and are not but a few pounds lighter.

Compare all of the specialty products in Bob's pantry with what is necessary for intermittent fasting. Bob's expensive boxes and cans of specialized diet products versus the intermittent fasting solution that requires you to simply "do nothing." That's right. In regard to food, you just do nothing. You don't eat. It doesn't cost you a dime. You actually save money in food you don't have to purchase for those meals. Intermittent fasting is **free, flexible, and simple.** Simple because intermittent fasting requires you to <u>not</u> do something instead of doing something. Dr. Jason Fung states in his books, "It is so simple that it can be explained in two sentences: Eat nothing. Drink water, tea, coffee, or bone broth". That's it. [4]

Compare this flexibility with other weight control programs. Intermittent fasting is done according to your own scheduling. It is flexible because it can be done at any time with any schedule and any duration. You can fast for sixteen hours, twenty-four hours, two days, six days, twenty-one days, or for as long as you want. You can fast using any diet: vegetarian, vegan, Keto, or Paleo. It can be done anywhere in the world. It doesn't matter. And if you don't feel well you can always stop fasting. You are in complete control.

Fasting is free because it doesn't require you to purchase anything. You simply stop doing something which is eating. And because your food consumption goes down, you'll actually be saving money at the grocery store. What a deal!

Another advantage, that patients note, is that intermittent fasting is a tool that gives them a sense of empowerment. They truly feel that they have taken back control of their healthcare. Psychologically, this greatly helps with their overall health picture because as the Bible says, "As a man thinks, so is he". Proper, mindful thinking is very healthy. It lowers cortisol levels (stress hormones), increases endorphin levels (feel good hormones), improves the overall physiology of the body, and helps with sleep. [5]

Everyday researchers and doctors are finding more and more benefits as a result of intermittent fasting. It's truly remarkable and we can only hope that the healthcare community can begin to embrace the benefits and accomplishments of intermittent fasting and really incorporate it as a viable and valuable modality of healthcare.

(1) Barnosky AR, Hoddy KK, Unterman TG, Varady KA.
"Intermittent fasting vs daily calorie restriction for type 2
diabetes prevention: a review of human findings."
Transl Res. 2014 Oct;164(4):302-11. doi:
10.1016/j.trsl.2014.05.013. Epub 2014 Jun 12.

(2) Goodrick C.L., Ingram D.K., Reynolds M.A., Freeman J.R., Cider
N.L., "Effects of Intermittent Feeding Upon Growth and Life Span
in Rats." Gerontology 1982;28:233–241
.

(3) https://www.healthline.com/nutrition/10-health-benefits-of-
intermittent-fasting

(4) Fung, Jason MD, "The Complete Guide to Fasting,"
2016, page 87

(5) Simon N. Young, PhD, "Biologic effects of mindfulness
meditation: growing insights into neurobiologic aspects of the
prevention of depression.",
J Psychiatry Neurosci. 2011 Mar; 36(2): 75–77.

(6) Sarah J. Mitchell, Michel Bernier, Julie A. Mattison, Miguel A.
Aon, Tamzin A. Kaiser, R. Michael Anson, Yuji Ikeno, Rozalyn M.
Anderson, Donald K. Ingram, Rafael de Cabo.
"Daily Fasting Improves Health and Survival in Male Mice
Independent of Diet Composition and Calories. "
Cell Metabolism, 2018; DOI: 10.1016/j.cmet.2018.08.011

CHAPTER 4 "Losing Weight"

By now you realize that Bob is big. No, I don't mean tall. He is round. His grandfather was a round guy and it seems that Bob is following in his footsteps. We can all agree that Bob needs to lose weight. We had a family gathering recently and after a passionate debate about theology the conversation turned to a perennial favorite. "What's the latest greatest diet plan to lose weight?" someone at the table asked, while intentionally avoiding Bob's eyes. It seems every family has a member who is trying to find ways to "fix" everyone's issues. Our family is no different. Although the question was not targeting Bob per se, everyone knew who the question was for. Putting down my fork, and also avoiding looking directly at Bob, I began to talk about intermittent fasting. Taking a quick peek at Bob I could see it in his eyes. "OH BOY, here we go again, another weight loss program." You might be thinking the exact same thing. Wronggggg!!!!!!! This is going to be totally different from anything you've ever read, studied or participated in.

Most of us have tried various weight loss programs throughout our lifetimes. Some have had some success but most programs have ended in failure. Dr. Jason Fung quite eloquently states in his book "The Obesity Code" that *"all diets work but all diets fail."*[1] Phil is one of my patients who has experienced this first hand. After years of trying every fad diet, his weight had ballooned to 330 pounds. He had lost varying amounts of weight over the years, but never had kept it off. Virtually all diets ultimately fail because the premise, of what actually causes obesity and then ultimately what causes weight loss, has been in error. The, "calories in – calories out" ---exercise more, paradigm has been proven to be wrong over and over. Having too much fat in the diet is also erroneous. So, it's going to take an understanding of a new paradigm of what is actually causing weight gain and then ultimately how we eliminate that weight. My experience, dealing with thousands of patients, has proven that this is not going to be an easy task. These original beliefs propagated by the healthcare industry for decades are not easily extinguished. They are simply just too ingrained in our culture. Phil was ready to make the leap. He began intermittent fasting while modifying the foods he eats. At the writing of this book Phil has lost eighty pounds and is well on the way to improved health. So, with Phil in mind, bear with me as I will begin to unpack, what I consider to be revolutionary, new information concerning weight loss.

It turns out that obesity is a problem of hormonal imbalance. Hormones are the central focus of understanding obesity, not calorie counting and such. Hormones tell us when we are hungry. Hormones tell us when we are full. Hormones tell us when to increase energy usage. Hormones tell us when to decrease energy usage. Our bodies are controlled by hormones. When it comes to obesity, there are primarily two hormones in question. They are **insulin** and **leptin.**

Insulin tells the body's cells to take glucose out of the blood and use it for energy. This occurs when we eat. Insulin is a hormone that also promotes the storage of fats and sugar. As a result, insulin, at sustained high levels, causes obesity. [2] Yes, **insulin causes obesity.** It's not calories. It's not fat. It's not laziness. Just insulin. This is easily provable in the mere fact that diabetic patients gain weight when given insulin. Insulin is like a gatekeeper to the cells of the body. When insulin levels are high, we store fat and sugar---- the gatekeeper (insulin) allows the fat and sugar to enter the cells. When insulin is low, we can then burn fat and sugar because the gatekeeper allows the body to empty the cells of excess sugar and fat.

Another factor is that the body's "set weight" is also controlled by hormones. [3] When insulin levels stay high, the body set weight continues to increase making it impossible to lose weight. *This is why lowering calories, while still eating regularly, doesn't work.* The insulin levels remain high even though calories are being lowered which doesn't allow sugar and fat burning to occur. Therefore, the set weight never gets a chance to reduce. The goal is to: lower insulin levels, lose the weight, reset the set weight, and then maintain the new weight.

Leptin is the second hormone that has to be addressed. Leptin is a hormone produced by the fat cells and contributes to satiety in a normal lean body. It tells the brain when we have had enough to eat. So, leptin and insulin perform opposite functions. Leptin reduces fat storage while insulin promotes fat storage.

In Bob and obese people this mechanism is all fouled up. Fasting blood levels of both insulin and leptin are elevated in obese people and the current thinking is that high insulin levels may actually inhibit the function of leptin therefore not allowing the brain to get the message to reduce fat storage and to stop eating. This will definitely put the weight on. When both of these levels remain high, it would indicate a state of both insulin and leptin resistance. The resistance occurs when the cells get overloaded with fat and sugar and are actually trying to protect themselves from damage. They simply can't and won't let anything else in. The higher sugar levels create a need for even higher levels of insulin trying to push more sugar into the cells. This creates even more resistance which eventually leads to more and more fat storage which equals obesity. [4] We are now set up for type 2 diabetes, because there is now nowhere for this overflow of sugar to go but into the bloodstream. Think of it this way. You have, let's say, a briefcase (a cell in the body) and you need to begin to place files (sugar molecules) into the briefcase for a meeting. As more and more files fill the briefcase it would begin to reach capacity and eventually it would be full and no more files would fit. But there are still files needed to be put in the briefcase. So, you (insulin) begin to jam more files into the briefcase. You may get a few more in there but now the briefcase is really full and there's absolutely no more room period. So now you use two hands (even more insulin than before) to try to push more files into the briefcase. The files begin to get dropped, spilling out their papers(sugar) all over the floor(bloodstream) generally making a mess. This is insulin resistance.

So, if hormonal imbalance, particularly insulin, is the cause of obesity then it would make sense that a therapeutic regimen must include a method to reduce insulin for a period of time, thereby allowing the hormonal picture to return back into balance. That method is intermittent fasting. It's not enough to just reduce calories. Intermittent fasting grants the body enough time to lower the insulin levels.

When we eat food, insulin spikes and blocks fat-burning and as a result the body resorts to burning the now available glucose from the food. If we continue to eat food on a regular basis the insulin levels continue to stay high. The high insulin levels keep the fats locked up in the cells making them unavailable to be burned. If stored fat cannot be burned, you cannot lose weight. Since insulin is a gatekeeper, we must lower the insulin levels long enough to allow the cells to be emptied of fat and sugar and then they can be burned. Insulin resistance on the other hand would hinder this process and often delay the ability to begin this process of cellular emptying. During insulin resistance, insulin levels may remain high for an extended period of time simply because the body is still in a mode of over producing insulin. Fasting is the only thing that will break this cycle.

Fasting begins the process of reversing obesity by first allowing the body to burn off the glycogen (stored sugar) in the liver. Once the glycogen levels begin to get low enough the body will begin to burn the stored levels of fat. This is all a result of the lower levels of insulin. And the longer the insulin stays at a lower level, the more the cells become insulin sensitive which decreases insulin resistance. The cells are then free to open up and dump their fat to be burned. It's that simple, but as mentioned before, it does take some time. It takes a long time to turn a big ship around. So, stay diligent. Keep your eye on the process and stay encouraged; it does work over time. To lose about one half of a pound per day is a reasonable expectation.

In closing this chapter, I would like to briefly mention one other hormone that is associated with obesity. Physiological or physical stress can release a hormone called cortisol. Cortisol causes weight gain. (5) This is provable by the fact that prednisone, a medicinal form of cortisol, causes weight gain when administered to patients. So, if you are under some form of stress; a stress management program should also be included as you fast.

(1) Fung, Jason MD. "The Obesity Code", 2016, page 215.

(2) UT Southwestern Medical Center. "High insulin levels tied to obesity pathway." ScienceDaily, 25 August 2014. www.sciencedaily.com/releases/2014/08/140825185319.htm

(3) Manfred J Müller, Anja Bosy-Westphal, Steven B Heymsfield, "Is there evidence for a set point that regulates human body weight?", F1000 Medicine Reports 2010 2:(59) (09 Aug 2010)

(4) Yazıcı D, Sezer H., "Insulin Resistance, Obesity and Lipotoxicity." Adv Exp Med Biol. 2017;960:277-304. doi: 10.1007/978-3-319-48382-5_12.

(5) Moyer AE, Rodin J, Grilo CM, Cummings N, Larson LM, Rebuffé-Scrive M., "Stress-induced cortisol response and fat distribution in women." Obes Res. 1994 May;2(3):255-62.

CHAPTER 5 "Diabetes"

Bob sat in his doctor's office listening as the results of a recent blood test were examined. "Well, you have a fatty liver and are pre-diabetic, Bob." His doctor reported. "You have to do something about this. Diabetes left untreated will dramatically shorten your life and lead to any number of miserable complications." Before the office visit was over Bob was prescribed a couple of prescriptions to try and reduce the blood sugar levels in his body. Blood sugar. It seems you can't live without it, yet too much will kill you. Poor Bob. Everyone is telling him that he has to do SOMETHING but no one is explaining to him what is actually going on in his body. If he could only see the high level of sugar coursing through his arteries. The small crystalline structures of glucose scuffing in arteries like sandblasting. His arteries are being damaged. Cholesterol is piled onto the damaged interior artery surfaces. Eventually the accumulated irritation and repairs is leading to permanent damage. Hardening of his arteries, the destruction of the fine arteries in his eyes, brain, nerves, and kidneys. Bob better do something fast or aging well won't even be the issue. Aging at all will become the question.

Diabetes is one of the major medical scourges of the day. In just 40 to 50 years diabetes has exploded to become a catastrophic epidemic. Huge amounts of money are spent every year on diabetes treatment as well as the many complications that occur as a result of the disease. How did this rarely-seen disease just one generation ago, now become such a problem. According to the Centers for Disease Control, more Americans are either diabetic or pre-diabetic than those that are not. That's shocking. Unfortunately, the great majority of these patients are overweight and will suffer complications as a result of their diabetic issues.

There are two types of diabetes, type 1 and type 2.

Type 1 diabetes is considered an autoimmune condition in which, for some reason, the beta cells of the pancreas are destroyed by the body's own immune system making it impossible for the pancreas to produce insulin. This is a life-threatening condition and must be treated with insulin injections.

Type 2 diabetes is, depending on who you consult, either a chronic progressive disease or a disease of diet and lifestyle. It is the body's response to constantly elevated blood sugar which results in high insulin levels ultimately leading to insulin resistance.

Insulin resistance means that the body loses its ability to respond to insulin's signal to allow sugar to enter the cells. The sugar now has nowhere else to go other than the bloodstream which equals type 2 diabetes.

Current medical treatment of type 2 diabetes consists of a kaleidoscope of different medications with more new ones on the horizon. When the initial medications fail, insulin is then introduced which is the same treatment used for type 1 diabetes. The problem is that the medications only help to control the blood sugar. They do not get to the underlying cause of the disease. Studies now show us that it can be done. [1]

So, what do we do? Well, if type 2 diabetes is a condition of excess sugar in the blood caused by the overload of the cells with glucose, then it would make sense to empty the cells of glucose. If the cells of the body weren't overloaded, then there would be no excess glucose in the bloodstream. Sound simple? It actually is. So how is this done?

 The first thing you have to do is quit putting glucose, and for that matter, fructose into the body. Obviously, this comes from consuming too many carbohydrates. All sugars are carbohydrates. But not all carbohydrates are sugar or will be converted to sugar.

Some carbohydrates are fiber which can be helpful. So, what is the first thing? Stop eating foods that are high in carbohydrates that are sugars or convert to sugar. Of course, the absolute best way to accomplish this is with fasting. Fasting not only eliminates sugar and carbohydrates, but all other foods that may be raising blood glucose and insulin levels.

The second thing you have to do is allow the body to eliminate the excess glucose hanging around in your system. Fasting is the most effective solution. When no new food is coming in, the body has no choice but to burn stored glucose and fat. The result is your blood sugar will come down. As the blood glucose levels stay at a consistently normal level you will no longer be considered diabetic. You have now successfully reversed your diabetes. At that point you would want to determine what would be the best way to maintain your new blood sugar levels. Obviously, a diet low in carbohydrates would be appropriate along with periods of intermittent fasting to keep the insulin levels at their new "set level".

Make sure to consult with your physician before starting any fasting, particularly if you're on any type 2 diabetes medications. Fasting will, more than likely, lower your blood glucose levels causing a need for less medication. You will then need your physician to monitor and make any necessary changes or adjustments to your dosages. You should monitor your blood glucose levels at least two to four times per day. And, obviously, if your sugar gets too low you must eat some sugar to bring your levels back to normal. Also don't forget to consult with your physician if you're on other non-diabetic related medications before fasting.

(1) E. L. Lim, K. G. Hollingsworth, B. S. Aribisala, M. J. Chen, J. C. Mathers, and R. Taylor
"Reversal of type 2 diabetes: normalisation of beta cell function in association with decreased pancreas and liver triacylglycerol."
Diabetologia. 2011 Oct; 54(10):2506–2514

CHAPTER 6 "Heart Health"

So, Bob went to his doctor to get a report on his lab work and lo and behold he was told, "you have high cholesterol and high triglycerides.'' "OMG!" Bob replied. "What am I gonna do?" Now the truth is Bob should have asked "What is high cholesterol and high triglycerides, and how does that affect me?"

 Instead, his doctor then summarily prescribed a statin drug to lower his cholesterol. As one of his friends once said, "Oh, I don't worry much about the stuff the doctor tells me. There is always a pill for that." Great! So now you have a choice to make as to whether you want to take the medication or take it upon yourself to improve your eating habits, start an exercise program or try to approach this from a more natural perspective. Let's take a look at the question Bob should have asked. "What is cholesterol and what does it matter?"

First of all, cholesterol is not a dirty word. Cholesterol is made in the liver and performs many vital functions in the body. It is a precursor to hormones, antibodies, and enzymes. It's neuroprotective, particularly in the brain. Cholesterol is an integral part of the cell membrane and helps with what enters and leaves the cells. Studies have shown that the more cholesterol you have in your brain, the less risk of dementia, depression and other neurological diseases. [1]

Cholesterol

The cholesterol number that you see in your blood work consists of primarily two components. They are HDL, which is considered the good cholesterol, and LDL, the bad cholesterol. There are others but these are the two biggies. The problem comes when you have too much of a particular part of the LDL component of cholesterol, the so-called bad cholesterol. There are two types of LDL particles, type A and type B. The culprit is the type B particles which are small and dense. These small oxidized particles contribute to plaque formation due to the availability of triglycerides and an inflammatory process that's occurring in the arterial walls. This is sort of like having sandpaper circulating around the bloodstream irritating the lining of the arteries. This sets you up for plaque formation leading to blockage in the arteries. Type A particles are large fluffy type particles and are generally harmless as they float around in the bloodstream. This is very interesting because a person could have a high LDL reading consisting of larger particles (type A) and not develop coronary artery disease. However, on the other hand, a person could have a low LDL reading with a high number of smaller particles (type B) and be at a higher risk of coronary artery disease. [2] This is super important when evaluating cardiovascular risk. Looking only at the LDL number, without knowing the type A and type B levels, would be incomplete information and could lead to improper treatment recommendations. So, when testing for cholesterol, your doctor should always order a particle size test. If not, you're not getting the full picture of your cardiovascular risk.

Triglycerides are another risk factor for heart disease. Triglycerides are formed in the liver when the glycogen levels become overloaded from eating too many carbohydrates. The liver converts the excess carbohydrates into triglycerides and then ships them out of the liver where they ultimately become LDL. Unfortunately, triglyceride levels in America are on the rise because of the increased consumption of carbohydrates. This is the story of Bob's life. The good news is that triglycerides can be controlled by low-carbohydrate diets and intermittent fasting because the liver will be slowed down in creating triglycerides.

Cholesterol, on the other hand, cannot be controlled by diet. The reason being is that 80 percent of cholesterol is made in the liver. So, diet makes very little difference in cholesterol levels. Nevertheless, the "low-fat mantra" still remains quite popular, even though multiple studies have confirmed that fat in the diet does not raise cholesterol. [3] If that's true, how can fasting lower cholesterol?

The answer goes back to the above explanation of how the excess glycogen in the liver begins to convert to triglycerides which is then transported out of the liver and ultimately becomes the so-called bad cholesterol LDL. LDL is a component of the total cholesterol number in your blood work. So if we can lower the LDL, we will lower the total cholesterol. The only way this can happen is to lower the production of triglycerides by the liver, which lowers the production of LDL, which then lowers the total cholesterol number. Intermittent fasting does this well. When fasting, triglycerides get lowered by default because of the lack of carbohydrates. And if you throw in some exercise, which increases HDL (the good cholesterol), you have a pretty significant plan of attack towards decreasing multiple cardiac risk factors. I love what doctor Jason Fung says in his book, The Complete Guide to Fasting, "For people worried about heart attacks and strokes, the question is not *Why are you fasting?* but *Why are you not fasting?*"[4] So heart health is obviously huge if we're going to age well.

(1) West R, Beeri MS, Schmeidler J, Hannigan CM, Angelo G, Grossman HT, Rosendorff C, Silverman JM.
"Better memory functioning associated with higher total and low-density lipoprotein cholesterol levels in very elderly subjects without the apolipoprotein e4 allele."
Am J Geriatr Psychiatry. 2008 Sep;16(9):781-5. doi: 10.1097/JGP.0b013e3181812790.

(2) Wolfson, Jack. "The Paleo Cardiologist." 2015; pp.13-15

(3) Michael Eades, Framingham Follies, "the blog of Doctor Michael R. Eades, M.D. ," September 26th, 2006, https://proteinpower.com/drmike/2006/09/26/framingham-follies/

(4) Fung, Jason. "The Complete Guide to Fasting." 2016, page 163

CHAPTER 7 "POLYCYSTIC OVARY SYNDROME (PCOS)

"Polycystic what?" Bob said as he overheard a conversation his wife was having on the phone. He just knew that the doctor had found something else wrong with him. "Butt out, Bob, this has nothing to do with you," his wife interrupted her phone call to set him straight. "Why not? The doctor says I am a mess. This is just one more straw on this fat camel's back," he retorted with a huff. "Take it from me, Bob. This is not about you unless you have sprouted ovaries overnight."

Through my years of practice, women with hormonal issues have presented, quite frequently, seeking a nutritional remedy to their issues. Hormonal issues affect all ages of women from very young girls all the way up into menopause and even beyond. A great majority of these hormonal problems respond very well to nutritional therapy. Some are just imbalances of the basic nutrition in the body, particularly iodine. Iodine is a very important activator of all hormones. Other women need glandular support with nutrients called protomorphogens. There are a variety of factors that commonly affect hormonal issues including stress, sugar, and the use of certain medications. But then there are the patients that don't respond so well.

Probably one of the most difficult, and at times, frustrating conditions that I see is when young girls and women present with a set of symptoms which include:

- Sudden onset of acne, especially in adulthood
- Increase central body weight gain
- Facial hair growth
- Irregular or no menstrual periods
- Loss of hair or male pattern baldness
- Difficulty getting pregnant due to ovulation problems

These are the symptoms of **polycystic ovary syndrome (PCOS).** This condition affects 1 in 10 women according to *women's health.gov* and is a real scourge to those that have it. If you have PCOS you could have all of these symptoms or different combinations of them. This particular syndrome is not only physically debilitating but is also emotionally difficult, especially for the women that are trying to get pregnant and can't. This can lead to additional issues of depression and hopelessness. Adding to the hopelessness is the fact that medical treatment has not been really successful. It consists of using birth control pills, Clomid (a drug that causes ovulation), and Metformin, (a medication used for type 2 diabetes). PCOS is generally regarded as incurable. Kind of a bleak picture.

To make the diagnosis of PCOS, you have two of the three following criteria:

1. Hyperandrogenemia, (too much Testosterone)
2. Polycystic ovaries
3. Anovulation, (few or no ovulatory menstrual cycles) (1)

Dr. Nadia Pateguana and Dr. Jason Fung gave an amazing lecture at the Low Carb Denver 2019 conference [1], in which they shed new light and hope on the subject of PCOS. They basically revealed that our old friend insulin, or too much of it, is the cause of PCOS. So, let's look at the process in which this occurs.

Hyperandrogenemia. Hyperandrogenemia means too much testosterone. It's too much testosterone that causes the facial and body hair, acne, and hair loss on the scalp, known as male pattern baldness. [2] So, where does all this testosterone come from? The answer is the ovaries and the adrenal glands. In the PCOS situation, the overproduction of testosterone is coming from the <u>ovaries not the adrenals</u>. The overproduction of testosterone is being caused by---

you guessed it--- hyperinsulinemia or again, too much insulin.

Another factor that goes hand-in-hand with the high testosterone issue is a substance called <u>sex hormone-binding globulin</u> (SHBG). SHBG is made in the liver and is supposed to bind free testosterone and keep it at a low-level thereby negating its effects on the body. [3] When SHBG is low, the free circulating testosterone becomes too high which then causes the hair growth, acne and so on. So here we go again. The culprit, is hyperinsulinemia that causes the low levels of SHBG. The high blood insulin levels cause the liver to decrease the production of SHBG. Here's a summary:

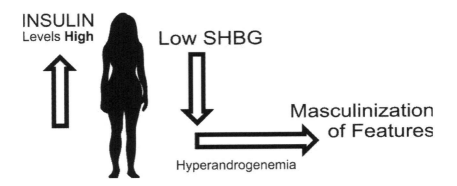

INSULIN
Levels **High**

Low SHBG

Masculinization of Features

Hyperandrogenemia

Polycystic Ovaries. The second aspect of the diagnosis of PCOS is polycystic ovaries. In a normal ovary during a normal menstrual cycle, the ovary produces an egg that ultimately gets released from the ovary and then meets up with the sperm. In PCOS, the eggs never mature because of a phenomenon called follicular arrest. [4] Follicular arrest occurs as a result of high insulin. These immature eggs are in fluid filled sacs called follicles. The follicles develop to a certain point and then stop at a pre ovulation level all because of high insulin. As a result, the follicles never develop and therefore cannot get out of the ovary as a normal egg. They are stuck at this pre ovulatory stage and since there's so many of them, the follicles begin to accumulate thereby forming cysts. Ovarian cysts come from these immature follicles. So again, it's too much insulin that's causing the follicular arrest, which is causing all of the cyst in the polycystic ovary.

Anovulation is the third criteria of the diagnosis and is pretty much self-explanatory from the previous paragraph. You are not going to ovulate if follicular arrest is occurring from high insulin levels. Here is an expanded diagram of the one above:

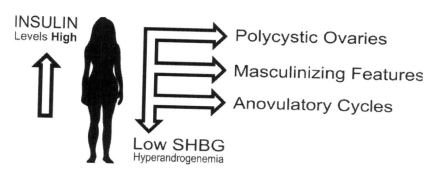

Other health problems have been associated with PCOS beyond the fertility issues which include, cardiovascular disease, type 2 diabetes, prediabetes, weight gain or obesity, insulin resistance, metabolic syndrome and probably many others.[5] When we drill down, we can see that all of these diseases have the commonality of being diseases of hyperinsulinemia. So, incredibly, it appears that high insulin is the cause of PCOS, its complications and all of its correlated diseases mentioned above.

So how do we treat PCOS? Well, if PCOS and all of its complications, are caused by hyperinsulinemia then it would make sense to treat it by lowering insulin. Birth control pills, fertility drugs nor antibiotics will lower insulin. However, these are the gold standard of medical treatment for PCOS and its complications. At present there is not a drug that will lower insulin that is safe. Therefore, I think it's obvious that the treatment is going to have to be something that gets to the root cause of hyperinsulinemia and lowers the insulin. And that something is our old champion, intermittent fasting along with low carbohydrate eating habits. All of these reduce insulin.

Through the years, I have also had great success at reducing ovarian cyst by the use of potassium iodide. The ovaries have the second highest concentration of iodine in the body. And beyond thyroid function, iodine promotes ovulation, activates hormones, promotes healthy detoxification of estrogen, plays a key role in immune function, and mitochondrial regulation. So, iodine should be added to the nutritional supplement regimen along with fasting and proper diet when treating PCOS. Just make sure you're monitoring your thyroid function when using iodine.

This whole PCOS thing, is just another breakthrough that has just blown my mind. I'm so grateful that doctors and researchers are bringing this information out into the open for the consumption of, not only the professionals, but for the general public as well. Once again, the research is catching up with all of the theories and opinions that didn't, until now, have good science behind it. This is just another step in the process of "Aging Well".

(1) HTTPS://IDMPROGRAM.COM/PCOS-LECTURE-FROM-LOW-CARB-DENVER/ ACCESSD JUNE 25, 2019.

(2) Alexiou E, Hatziagelaki E, Pergialiotis V, Chrelias C, Kassanos D, Siristatidis C, Kyrkou G, Kreatsa M, Trakakis E. "Hyperandrogenemia in women with polycystic ovary syndrome: prevalence, characteristics and association with body mass index." Horm Mol Biol Clin Investig. 2017 Mar 1;29 (3):105-111.
 doi: 10.1515/hmbci-2016-0047.

(3) Chandrika N Wijeyaratne; SA Dilini Udayangani; Adam H Balen. "Ethnic-specific Polycystic Ovary Syndrome." Expert Rev Endocrinol Metab. 2013;8(1):71-79.

(4) Jonard S, Dewailly D.
"The follicular excess in polycystic ovaries, due to intra-ovarian hyperandrogenism, may be the main culprit for the follicular arrest." Hum Reprod Update. 2004 Mar-Apr;10(2):107-17.

(5) https://jeanhailes.org.au/health-a-z/pcos/complications, accessed June 23, 2019.

CHAPTER 8 "Inflammation"

Bob was sitting in his underwear. The paper of the exam table crinkled and made noise as he scooted around to get comfortable. He dutifully has appeared on the appointed day for his annual physical exam. He knew what was coming. "Bob, you're obese. When are you going to do something about this?" But this year Bob had a few questions to ask his GP. "Doctor, I have noticed these hard-knobby spots developing on the knuckles of my fingers," Bob said holding up his hands. The doctor took all of three seconds to deliver the bad news. "These are early signs of developing arthritis." Arthritis! I'm too young to have arthritis!

Arthritis, psoriasis, rheumatoid arthritis, and fibromyalgia are all types of inflammation inside the body. Inflammation has become a pretty hot topic these days as more people are being diagnosed with one of these painful and at times debilitating diseases. And I think it fits appropriately in the context of the subjects of intermittent fasting and how to "age well". No serious discussion concerning health would be complete without addressing inflammation. Inflammation has obviously been around forever but the winds are changing in how to treat it and what causes it. No longer can health professionals just blow off these conditions as being "idiopathic"; that is "we don't know where it comes from or how it was contracted." Then the doctor says, "You'll just have to live with it". The same goes for treatment regimens, which are basically trying to deal with the symptoms and often have their own side effect issues. While symptomatic relief is necessary at times, it should not be the end goal. Research is now too extensive and credible to not pursue additional therapeutic models.

The inflammation that I am referring to is not the inflammation that is short term, such as a wound that is healing, a sprained joint or a short-term illness. I'm referring to the chronic or long term sustained type of inflammation that never resolves, like the chronic conditions mentioned above. This type of inflammation, if around long enough, begins to take on a life of its own and can ultimately trigger dreaded autoimmune diseases. This is where the body's immune system can no longer distinguish between attacking the body's normal cells or bad cells. Unfortunately, we all know someone that has an autoimmune condition and just how devastating it can be. When I was in chiropractic school, we were taught that if you had anything autoimmune, it was tough luck. We didn't have a clue as to what caused it and even knew less about how to treat it other than blast it with prednisone. That, fortunately, has changed.

We now know a lot about the genesis of chronic sustained inflammation. They include, *inflammatory foods, overgrowth of gut bacteria, nutritional deficiencies, mitochondrial malfunction, hormonal issues, toxic overload of chemicals, pesticides, drugs and heavy metals.* I'm sure there are others but knowing what we know now, there is no excuse for clinicians to not pursue therapeutic protocols that could and would possibly heal these "incurable" diseases instead of the present standard of care.

Inflammatory Foods

In my practice we have, for many years, been advocates of the paleo and ketogenic diet as a start towards reducing inflammation. This fits in perfectly with the lifestyle eating protocols that parallels intermittent fasting and the treatment of hyperinsulinemia. The resulting conditions of hyperinsulinemia, such as type 2 diabetes, fatty liver, cardiovascular disease, polycystic ovary syndrome, as well as all the other conditions mentioned in this book, are inflammatory diseases.[1] So as we implement intermittent fasting, as a treatment for hyperinsulinemia, we are going to automatically begin to reduce and wipeout chronic inflammation.[2] So it's important to eat good non-inflammatory foods when pursuing health and longevity. Gluten, sugar, cow's milk and ice cream are all highly inflammatory type foods, and must be avoided. After all of that, certain people will still have specific allergies to some foods that are good foods. I have actually seen people that were allergic to almonds for example. At that point we have to do some special testing to identify these foods and eliminate them from the diet as well.

Overgrowth of Gut Bacteria

SIBO (small intestinal bacterial overgrowth) is another highly inflammatory situation that occurs in the intestinal tract. [3] This occurs when the ratio of good bacteria and bad bacteria get out of balance. This causes inflammation in the gut that usually results in a situation called *leaky gut*. Leaky gut allows undigested foods, bacteria, and other digestive components to leak through the gut wall back into the bloodstream and lymphatics. This causes inflammatory issues throughout the body, particularly in the brain because the immune system now has to attack these unwanted invaders. Antimicrobial herbs and probiotics have been effective in restoring the gut back to normal health however, it may require some other nutritional intervention as well. Intermittent fasting and proper foods are also very helpful. [4]

Nutritional Deficiencies

Nutritional deficiencies are pretty self-explanatory as a cause of inflammation. Vitamins, minerals, enzymes, coenzymes, etc. are involved in many biochemical and physiological functions and processes. If these nutrients become deficient or if their ratios get altered the body will have a response. The response could be in the form of inflammation. It could affect a number of systems including the immune system, cardiovascular system, digestion, brain function, or musculoskeletal system. For this reason, we want to have a protocol that provides good nutrient coverage.

Mitochondrial Dysfunction

Mitochondrial dysfunction is characterized primarily in three ways. 1) Impaired ATP production (the way energy is made in the cell), 2) increased free radical production which damages cells, 3) increased inflammation. [5] Mitochondria are the little energy makers inside of almost every cell in the body. The science is pretty clear that the health of the mitochondria is of utmost importance. In other words, unhealthy mitochondria lead to an unhealthy cell, which leads to an unhealthy body triggering an inflammatory response. This inflammation can occur anywhere at any time in the body but the good news is that intermittent fasting is an excellent modality for rebooting and reprogramming the mitochondria back to a position of health.

Hormonal Issues

Hormones are very powerful substances in the body causing and reacting to all kinds of phenomena, for example, female hormones flowing in the various phases of the menstrual cycle or the thyroid hormones as they relate to metabolism. We all know what happens when these hormones get out of balance. It's usually not a very pretty picture. How about the hormone insulin, a major subject of this book, which can progress to hyperinsulinemia with all of its resultant problems being discussed in other chapters *(see chapter on PCOS).* All of these different hormones create imbalances that create inflammation in their own right.

Toxic Overload

Toxins that accumulate in the body from chemicals, pesticides, heavy metals, drugs and their residues, and organic pollutants cause massive inflammation.

We are literally in a war caused by the onslaught of toxins from many directions including our foods, air, water, industrial, and environmental pollutants. These offenders tend to take their effect upon the mitochondria of the cells. As a result, the mitochondria now become compromised in their ability to produce energy. This can cause the cells to become insulin resistant as well as create a compromised immune system. This generates an overall cellular failure and the body will begin to respond with inflammation to deal with the compromised cells. Chemicals, pesticides, drugs and their residues are more fast acting, while heavy metals tend to accumulate over a period of time and then begin to manifest into some type of ailment. Therefore, it becomes very important that we immediately implement a program of avoidance and then detoxification so that we can protect and preserve the mitochondrial function not to mention the fact that we'll feel much better as well. Prolonged exposure to toxins really debilitates the body's ability to "age well" and can very likely precipitate into some very serious diseases. We must really watch and evaluate what we eat, breathe, drink and what we're being exposed to environmentally.

(1) Carl de Luca and Jerrold M. Olefsky.
"Inflammation and Insulin Resistance."
FEBS Lett. 2008 Jan 9; 582(1): 97–105.

(2) Faris MA, Kacimi S, Al-Kurd RA, Fararjeh MA, Bustanji YK,
Mohammad MK, Salem ML.
"Intermittent fasting during Ramadan attenuates proinflammatory
cytokines and immune cells in healthy subjects."
Nutr Res. 2012 Dec;32(12):947-55. doi:
10.1016/j.nutres.2012.06.021. Epub 2012 Oct 4.

(3) Ricci JER Júnior, Chebli LA, Ribeiro TCDR, Castro ACS, Gaburri PD,
Pace FHDL, Barbosa KVBD, Ferreira LEVVDC, Passos MDCF, Malaguti
C, Delgado ÁHDA, Campos JD, Coelho AR, Chebli JMF.
"Small-Intestinal Bacterial Overgrowth is Associated With Concurrent
Intestinal Inflammation But Not With Systemic Inflammation in
Crohn's Disease Patients."
J Clin Gastroenterol. 2018 Jul;52(6):530-536. doi:
10.1097/MCG.0000000000000803.

(4) Marlene Remely, Berit Hippe, Isabella Geretschlaeger, Sonja
Stegmayer, Ingrid Hoefinger, andAlexander Haslberger.
"Increased gut microbiota diversity and abundance of
Faecalibacterium prausnitzii and Akkermansia after fasting: a pilot
study."
Wien Klin Wochenschr. 2015; 127(9-10): 394–398.

(5) Vasquez,Alex DC ND DO.
"Inflammation Mastery," 4th edition. 2004, page 623

CHAPTER 9 "Nutrition"

It's 3 o'clock in the morning. Bob is sound asleep snuggled under his covers with his wife on the opposite side of the bed, and their three dogs gently snoring between them. Another night in paradise - or so it would seem. But Bob had spent the day outside working in the hot Florida sun. "Sweating like a pig" hardly describes the fluid loss he experienced. Now Bob knows about dehydration and fluid replacement so he had been drinking water throughout the day and into the evening. What he didn't know was that his body was suffering from mineral depletion. Out with the sweat came important minerals such as potassium, calcium and magnesium. So, in the wee hours of the night, his calf muscle suddenly spasms. The pain shoots through his body an unsolicited scream erupts from his voice. The pain is unbearable and suddenly his wife and all three dogs have been jarred from their sleep. The entire house has been disrupted all because Bob's body has depleted some basic minerals that are necessary for it to function well.

When I review all of the studies, books, and articles concerning intermittent fasting, I see very little written on the importance of nutritional supplementation as part of the plan. When we begin

' intake, I think it is crucial that we
ic levels of vitamins, minerals, oils,
It becomes even more important as
ds are lengthened. The longest fast in
days, was maintained with
nutritional supplementation. Nutrients are essential
for proper physiological and hormonal function. If
nutrients are lacking, the body cannot function
normally and ultimately will result in disease. It makes
no sense to accumulate all of the benefits of
intermittent fasting on one hand and then lose them
as a result of developing a nutritional deficiency on
the other.

There are certain *basic* nutrients that are needed to
maintain a good nutritional status while fasting. They
include:

1. A complete whole food multivitamin supplement
2. A multimineral supplement
3. A complete and balanced fatty acid supplement
4. Coenzyme Q10
5. Sea Salt

Beyond the basics, there are other nutrients that
could be important depending on the clinical
condition of the patient including: Lipoic Acid, Vitamin
D3, probiotics, Vitamin C, additional magnesium,

iodine, resveratrol, Vitamin E, additional B vitamins, and certain amino acids. The need of these additional supplements would be determined by either lab work or through an energetic method such as Contact Reflex Analysis or Applied Kinesiology.

Let's look at some of the benefits that the above five mentioned **basic** nutrients provide:

Multivitamin supplement--- Offers a good start at covering the basics for our overall nutritional needs. Multiple clinical studies have shown that multivitamin use, improves nutritional status and reduces the risk for chronic disease. It begins to fill in the nutritional gaps that are left as a result of nutrient deficiencies found in foods today.

Multimineral supplement--- Many multivitamin supplements, including the good ones, often lack a sufficient mineral load, particularly the trace minerals. This is why they are added to the recommendations. Minerals offer a multitude of benefits--- too numerous to include in this writing--- but I think most would agree that proper levels are crucial for biochemical efficiency leading to optimal health. One aspect I do want to address is the importance that minerals play in the hydration process of the body. I would say that when you mention hydration to most people, they would immediately reply that it is the amount of fluid that you drink. That is only partially true. The fact of the matter is that there's two other components that are required for good hydration levels. Minerals and salt (sea salt) are those components. Salt will be explained shortly. The minerals help to manage fluid distribution throughout the body. Think of them as traffic cops managing traffic---you go here, you go there, don't go there, etc. Without minerals, the fluid either goes right through you (urinating all the time after drinking) or it ends up in places it doesn't belong, such as the hands, feet, legs or belly (so called beer belly). We want the fluids we drink to end up in the tissue where it can properly perform normal functions. It's the minerals that make it happen.

Complete and Balanced Fatty Acid supplement---This would include *fish oil, flaxseed oil, borage oil,* which contains *ALA, EPA, DHA, GLA, and oleic acid.* Again, the benefits are numerous, including an anti-inflammatory effect, enhances insulin sensitivity (good for hyperinsulinemia), is cardio-protective (protects the heart), lubricates the joints, is a hormone precursor, has an antioxidant effect, has a mitochondria (energy producing organelles within most cells of the body) protective effect, and many more.

Coenzyme Q10---Crucial nutrient for proper muscle function in the heart and in the skeletal muscle, especially as we get older. It also has an anti-inflammatory effect, helps with blood sugar control, reduces blood insulin levels, and is crucial for mitochondrial energy production. Normal mitochondrial function is vital to the human condition. Without it life doesn't exist. Consequently, sick or corrupted mitochondria cause many conditions and diseases. Sugar and hyperinsulinemia, sizeable subjects of this book, are two of the major corrupting culprits that inhibits cellular function and by default the mitochondria which then begins the pathway to disease. There are many other offenders including toxins, pesticides, and heavy metals as well. Therefore, the protection and enhancement of the function of the mitochondria is super important. Coenzyme Q10, lipoic acid, and the above-mentioned oils are all very good nutrients that enhance mitochondrial function and protection.

Sea Salt---Crucial in the hydrating process of the body. It is one of the three components of hydration, fluid and minerals being the other two. Salt along with magnesium can, at times, get too low during intermittent fasting and needs to be supplemented. Salt also maintains blood volume and blood pressure to ensure that blood carrying oxygen gets to the cells and tissues of the body. There's a lot of misconceptions and confusion concerning salt due to erroneous research that was conducted in the 1950s. The resultant "salt scare" that came from this research quickly caught on as a cause of high blood pressure and other cardiovascular problems despite the lack of any scientific backing and continues today. Multiple Studies have now been conducted that has debunked the concerns with salt. [1] Bob could alleviate his late night "Charlie horses" just by including sea salt in his diet, especially after a long day in the hot sun.

At this point, there is a very important aspect of nutritional supplementation that must be discussed. You see, the source of nutritional supplementation cannot be over- emphasized because how and where supplements are made are crucial as to their effectiveness. Unfortunately, many store-bought supplements are synthetically made in laboratories. I can't tell you how many times patients bring bags of supplements to my office; and when I examine and research them, they turn out to be virtually worthless. You have to be very careful, particularly with the oils, as we find many are already rancid at the time of purchase due to faulty processing. You want to purchase supplements that are made from organic foods. While not every single component in a supplement can be natural and organic, we want to find the supplement companies that have the highest percentage of organic whole foods as possible. Our bodies are made to run on whole foods not chemicals made in a laboratory. In fact, synthetic vitamins can often do harm in the body in high enough doses.

For these reasons, our office carries only the highest-grade supplements on the market, because when we make nutritional recommendations, we want to give your body the highest odds of obtaining a therapeutic result. If you would like to know the specific products and companies referred to in this chapter, please contact our office at 321-452-6264.

Another reason for the need of supplementation is the fact that foods today often times have decreased nutritional value. Even organic foods are suspect at times. This is because a lot of the soils, that fruits and vegetables are grown in are deficient in nutrients themselves due to over utilization and bad farming techniques. Once again, where you get your foods are very important. In my opinion, aging well is going to require nutrient supplementation.

(1)Alderman, M. H., H. Cohen,and S. Madhavan.
"Dietary sodium intake and mortality: the National Health
and Nutrition Examination Survey (NHANES I)."
The Lancet. 1998 Mar 14;351(9105):781-5.

CHAPTER 10 "Complications & Plateaus"

Beginning a regimen of fasting, is often very simple. It can be as easy as just skipping a meal, then proceeding on to increased times between eating. Suddenly you are losing weight. But our bodies are resilient and want to hold onto resources, even if it is just excess fat.   These are the times when the body will actually resist the process as changes are being made to the types of foods we are eating and the intervals between eating those foods. This resistance can manifest itself in many different forms. In this section we are going to identify the most common complications and plateaus that occur during a fast and then offer solutions to those situations.

I just can't do it!

The first obstacle that usually occurs is that many people have the belief that they cannot fast. This belief comes from a myriad of reasons and fears. This would include: "Oh I will starve", or "My blood sugar will drop, I'll get headaches, my schedule won't permit it, my spouse won't cooperate, I just love to eat, I'm a sugar addict" and so on. The truth of the matter is that fasting is really quite easy once people are properly informed and given the proper support and encouragement.

The first few days are always the hardest and will often require some adjustment. The first thing that pops up is usually hunger. Hunger is an interesting subject. Many experts believe that hunger starts in the mind and that there's actually a conditioned response to eating on certain schedules. "Classical conditioning" is big in the psychology world (think of Pavlov's dog) also known as behaviorism.[1] We wake up at 7 a.m.---it's time to eat--- we come home from work--- it's time to eat---we go to the movies---where's the popcorn? Intermittent fasting is a great way to break this conditioned response. It just takes a little time to allow our bodies to be reconditioned to a new way of eating and how we actually think about it. This phenomenon has been very interesting to watch in my practice. I have seen some of the most hard-core resistance turn into the most fanatical proponents. I personally think it is how they now actually see that intermittent fasting is different. It's not just another diet program. The insulin reduction issue, once they see it, is the difference from other diet plans they've tried in the past. And the science behind it just makes sense for a change.

Snacking

Snacks are another problem when it comes to conquering hunger. This is often the place we run to when we're hungry. Personal experience has shown that replacing the habit of snacking with a cup of bulletproof coffee, a cup of tea or a small spoon of a nut butter (cashew or almond) is effective. This is because of the satiating effect of the fat content. Once again it will take a little reconditioning to get out of some of the bad habits. Replacing meals with bulletproof coffee works as well for the same reason. Bulletproof coffee contains heavy whipping cream, MCT oil and butter, lots of fat. Finding ways to stay active on fasting days, is another technique that helps you get through the fast. In the end though, you will ultimately have to just hang tough and press through. The good news is that many of my patients have reported that hunger only lasts through the second day of the fast. After that it gets much easier as hunger actually subsides. This is contrary to the belief of many, that hunger ramps up and gets increasingly stronger the further you get away from a meal. Studies show that this is simply not true.

Hormones

There is also a hormonal aspect of hunger. The hormone ghrelin causes a spike in the hunger response. Studies have shown that the spike that ghrelin causes is temporary and oftentimes can be pushed through. How many times have we been busy with some sort of project and actually worked through a meal? Then a couple of hours pass and we've forgotten that we were hungry, so we just push on through till the next meal. The effect of ghrelin disappears relatively quickly and, by knowing this, will help us to persevere.

Other complications and concerns that may occur during fasting would include:

Muscle cramps
Fatigue
Heartburn
Dizziness
Headaches
Constipation
Irritability
Growling digestion [1]

Let's address them one at a time.

Muscle Cramps

Muscle cramps are usually caused by either a lack of minerals or salt (sea salt). In my office, we use an analytical technique called Contact Reflex Analysis (CRA), taught by Dr. Dick Versendaal DC, that uses reflex points on the acupuncture meridian system to determine if indeed there is a mineral or salt deficiency. If CRA reveals a deficiency then appropriate recommendations are made. Hydration is also an important consideration and has to be balanced with salt and minerals. If you do not have the availability of this modality of testing then you will have to make sure you have enough minerals and salt in your diet, particularly magnesium, along with being well hydrated.

Fatigue

Fatigue is not typically an issue, in fact, many people report an increase in energy during fasting. You should be able to work and perform your daily functions as normal. If you should have persistent fatigue while fasting you should stop and seek medical advice.

Heartburn

Heartburn can be caused by a hiatal hernia. This is when the stomach gets forced up into the diaphragm which is the big muscle that separates the abdominal area from the chest and lung area. We have a technique in our office that we use to pull the stomach down into its normal position if indeed you have this problem. Many chiropractors and other physicians around the country have been trained in this technique. If you don't have someone at your disposal that can administer this treatment then you would have to resort to other remedies many of which can be found on the internet. Lack of digestive enzymes could be another cause of heartburn and could be helped with supplemental digestive enzymes. Persistent heartburn however should be checked out medically.

Dizziness

In our office we find that dizziness is most often caused by dehydration. Most people don't realize that dehydration is a three-legged stool. In order to be properly hydrated, all three legs have to be addressed. The first leg, obviously, is that we must have enough fluid in our body. The second leg is that we must have enough salt in our body. We recommend sea salt because it contains trace minerals and electrolytes. The third leg is that we have to have enough minerals in our body because minerals are the traffic cops that direct fluid to the proper places in the body. If we don't have this fluid management, we either lose the fluid too quickly through urination or the body tends to store it in the wrong places such as the belly, hands, legs or feet. We always recommend a multi-mineral supplement when fasting. Medications are notorious for causing dizziness as well and these should be monitored and possibly adjusted by the physician that prescribed them.

Headaches

Headaches are one of the most common complaints particularly early on during the fast. We have found that dehydration again can be the culprit. Our previously mentioned CRA testing has confirmed this and oftentimes reveals that it is a lack of salt. So, using extra sea salt would be appropriate. Coffee containing caffeine works as well. This was particularly helpful to me personally. Organ congestion, which can back-up toxins into the body can also cause headaches. CRA or Applied Kinesiology again can help identify these problems. More on this below.

Constipation

Because we are eating less food, naturally we're going to have fewer bowel movements. Increasing fiber will help and we like to use magnesium as a laxative if necessary. As long as you're not experiencing any discomfort there is not too much to worry about. Remember to stay well hydrated and if any problems present themselves, then seek professional help.

Irritability

Irritability is generally not a problem with intermittent fasting. Many people think that it is a state of mind or could possibly be other emotional problems below the surface. I think that once we acquiesce to the fact that we're going to begin a potential life changing program, it puts us into a better frame of mine, thus less irritability.

Growling Digestion

We recommend a nutrition called Super Phosphozyme made by Biotics Research Corporation. This is a liquid ortho phosphoric acid which is mainly the mineral phosphorus. Two or three droppers full in some water seems to settle the stomach and digestive tract. If this is not available some sea salt in water will usually work.

Other Problems to be Aware Of

Diabetics need to be monitored closely. If you are taking insulin you should monitor your blood sugar three to four times per day. If you become unstable, shaky or sweaty, immediately take your blood sugar and adjust accordingly. Make sure you keep your doctor informed so that he or she can make changes to your medication if necessary.

Blood pressure should be monitored as well. You can refer to the above information concerning dizziness, and you will want to monitor your electrolytes and minerals.

If you have any persistent nausea, vomiting, high or low blood pressure, lethargy, or fatigue, you should stop your fasting and consult your doctor. These symptoms are not consistent with intermittent fasting and could be a warning of something more serious.

Plateaus

Twenty years ago, Bob went on the Atkins low carb diet for six months and lost 40 pounds. He was in his early forties and the pounds seemed to fall away. Eventually, he hit a plateau where he stopped losing weight. He became frustrated and after a few weeks of no progress, he quit the diet. Losing the weight was a good thing for Bob. But it was just a diet to him and you know Bob and pizza (hi-carbs), soon he was back to eating poorly. Now, many years later, after numerous other diet attempts, he is up seventy pounds! Losing a little weight is somewhat easy, but the emotional frustration of hitting plateaus is destructive to diets leading to failure and relapse.

This is the marvel of intermittent fasting. It is not a diet. Hitting a plateau is also common in intermittent fasting. Plateaus occur when, for some reason, our progress seems to halt, despite the fact that we're doing exactly what we've been doing all along. This would include mainly weight loss but not limited to other improvements that we may be experiencing as well. Some plateaus are very easy to fix and some are more complicated. Experiences, in our office, tells us that the simplest thing to do is to change the amount of time that we are fasting. In other words, if we are doing a 24-hour intermittent alternating day fast, we could increase our fasting time to 36 hours or if we were doing a 16 hour fast, we might increase it to 24 hours. Most of the time this will be effective. However, in our practice, we have found a few other issues that can lend itself to a plateaued situation.

I always like to evaluate whether a person has a congested organ, particularly the organs of elimination such as the liver, gallbladder, kidneys, and urinary bladder. As we lose weight, all of the byproducts of weight loss have to be eliminated through these organs. If they become overloaded and congested then the process will certainly be slowed if not halted. This will, potentially, cause a recycling of toxins back into the body creating other issues including congested sinuses, congested bronchioles, skin rashes, headaches, and just an overall lousy feeling. In fact, these symptoms could be an early sign that a plateau could be coming or is already in progress. If these congested organs are not addressed the plateau would continue no matter what other remedies you may try. So how do we deal with a congested organ?

Contact Reflex Analysis is an excellent modality to identify congested organs by testing their corresponding reflex points. Blood work is also effective but usually doesn't show problems in the organs until much later. Once an organ is identified as being congested, it has to be flushed or cleansed. There are basically two ways to flush an organ. You can use one of the many herbal organ flushing programs that are on the market or you can use a manual flushing process that has to be implemented by someone that is trained in visceral manipulation and organ flushing. This is the method that I prefer in our practice. It's quicker, easier and there's not as much discomfort that's often seen with the herbal flushes. Once the organ has been opened up, you'll be back on track and able to continue with your fast.

Another plateau condition that we've seen in our office, even though it's rare, is when the body seems to want to detoxify at a very high rate and as a result will slow down or halt progress. It's commonly known that the body stores toxins in the fatty tissues of the body. As we begin to burn off fat and lose weight these toxins are released into the body and have to be eliminated. Some of these toxins are of a nasty variety including pesticides, petroleum residues, plastics, cleaning chemicals, and heavy metals. If the body's elimination of these toxins is hindered in any way, then we have to slow down and maybe even use some special supplementation to remove these toxins before resuming the fast.

Always remember that you can break your fast if you feel unwell for any reason. You can always start your fast when you start to feel well again. Always listen to your body and seek medical attention when needed.

(1) Wolpe J, Plaud JJ.
"Pavlov's contributions to behavior therapy. The obvious and not so obvious."
Am Psychol. 1997;52(9):966-72.

(2) yahoo.com/lifestyle/9-common-side-effects-intermittent-013529487.html, accessed June 23 2019.

CHAPTER 11 "Can Everyone Fast?"

The answer is no. Because of their physiological and psychological makeup, some people should simply refrain from fasting. Others may have a disease that would make it too risky to fast.

You should not fast if:

- You're pregnant
- You're breastfeeding
- You have an eating disorder such as anorexia
- You're under 18 years old. (However, in some cases of obesity, it wouldn't hurt for a child to skip some meals to get insulin levels down. Always check with your doctor first.)
- Certain diseases such as kidney disease, or gout
- You have a severe nutritional deficiency
- You're underweight
- You have type 1 diabetes
- You have gastroesophageal reflux disease

Pregnant and breastfeeding women need to maintain a good nutritional regimen for proper fetal development and child development after birth. The mother must remain healthy as all of the baby's nutrition will be coming from the mother.

People with anorexia definitely have no business fasting as they are usually already underweight and malnourished. They actually need to be eating and will probably need some psychological help as well.

Any kind of disease involving an organ should be cleared by a doctor before attempting any fasting. These organs need to be evaluated and do not need any additional stress.

Being underweight speaks for itself as these people need to be eating however, if they're chronically underweight, they need to be evaluated to determine what is the cause.

Some type 1 diabetic patients do some fasting but it would need to be done under very close supervision of a physician. You don't want to go into ketoacidosis, which is too many ketone bodies in the blood. This could be life threatening.

Gastroesophageal reflux disease (GERD) is a touchy situation. Sometimes fasting can make things worse as there's no food in the stomach to absorb the acid production. However, losing weight often helps GERD. So, proceed with caution. One approach is to slowly and incrementally experiment with some intermittent fasting and see how it works. If heartburn returns then discontinue fasting and seek treatment to resolve the GERD then you can proceed with fasting.

The main thing to always remember is that if you are feeling bad in anyway, you must stop fasting immediately and contact your healthcare provider.

CHAPTER 12 "Our Quest for the Longevity Lifestyle"

Okay so here we are. This is where we're going to put it all together and show you how to actually implement intermittent fasting in conjunction with eating whole foods for the purpose of "aging well". We're going to start off with a brief review of the material related to intermittent fasting, insulin, insulin resistance, and blood sugar. Then we'll finish out with the actual implementation recommendations and how to eat on feeding days.

 As previously stated, history has shown that most diets work in the short run, but over time they ultimately fail. Why is this? Let's take weight gain for instance. Permanent weight loss requires that we start with a short-term solution, usually a diet, but then the longer-term solution requires that we address the hormonal aspects of the condition particularly hyperinsulinemia (too much insulin in the blood). This would also include most diseases in general not discounting the fact that there's other factors involved such as age, gender, smoking, excessive alcohol use, stress, etc. Pursuing the hormonal "reset" will contribute greatly to actually keeping weight off permanently as well as enhancing our health in general. What do I mean by this term *reset?*

Our bodies in general and its systems specifically, like to resist change. To make it simple, imagine that of all the systems in our body, whether it's hormonal or otherwise, have a thermostat like the one in your house. If, for example our weight goes up or goes down, the systems of the body will cause it to revert to its original weight. This is caused by the hypothalamus gland located just beneath the brain. If I have my house thermostat set at 75 degrees and then go open all the doors and let the 90-degree outside air enter, it will warm up the house. However, when I close the doors the air conditioning will bring the house back down to 75 degrees. The same thing happens with insulin. As we age, resistance to insulin increases to a new "set level" which makes it more difficult to not only lose weight but to keep it off as well. This is exactly why losing weight is so frustrating. But if we were to do something (intermittent fasting) to change the thermostat setting of the house we could then affect a permanent change to the temperature (weight and many other ailments). That change is brought about when we address the condition of hyperinsulinemia with fasting. We have seen that throughout this book. While disease remains multifactorial, the common uniting theme is the hormonal imbalance of hyperinsulinemia.[1] **This is the major breakthrough.** This is the key point to be remembered. While the concept of fasting has been around for thousands of years, Dr. Jason Fung, in his book, *The Complete Guide to Fasting,* has, in my opinion, taken the lead in bringing this subject into a more user-friendly form. There are others but his knowledge and passion for this subject has been inspiring.

So how do we "reset" the body to attain our goals of good health as well as weight loss and other health issues? Well, if hyperinsulinemia is the problem, then it would make sense that lowering insulin would go a long way towards accomplishing these goals. In the next chapter, I will outline the process in which these goals can be accomplished.

(1)Fung, J., The Obesity Code, 2016, page 218

CHAPTER 13 "How to Get Started"

In my clinical practice there are two main questions that are always asked when diet or fasting are mentioned. "What am I supposed to eat?" and, "when am I supposed to eat it?" Fasting, whether it's in the intermittent form or of a more prolonged form, has been the missing element in this quest for good health, weight loss, and lowering high levels of insulin.

Let's start with fasting---the **when.** While there are many renditions out there, my definition of fasting is *a period of time that food is restricted and allows only non-caloric drinks.* The allowable drinks would include water, tea, black coffee, coffee with heavy whipping cream and organic bone broth. Sugar, honey, fructose, agave nectar, maple syrup, and other sugars are prohibited. Juice fasting is not permitted because of the sugar content. In our practice we have found that the ability to drink coffee during the fasting days has helped with headaches that occur when in the early stages of a fast. Bulletproof coffee helps as well due to the fact that it contains fats that help with hunger. The fats, in the coffee, do <u>not</u> affect insulin levels. They also decrease cravings and seems to help mental clarity.

Staying hydrated through the fast is a priority. Starting each day with an 8 oz glass of water is a good plan and I personally like to add a little bit of lemon juice and even some sea salt to the water. This makes the water more absorbable as well as improving the taste. Continue to drink water throughout the day. Having enough trace minerals in the body is also important in the hydration issue and was explained in more detail in the chapter on nutrition.

When am I supposed to eat?
All types of fasting are effective, the key is to find the right one that works best for your situation. What may work for one person may not work for another. **Intermittent Fasting** consist of alternating periods of eating and then not eating. Fasting times can range from as little as 12 hours all the way up to 30-40 days and fasting times can be switched around. Based on multiple sources, I think a 24-hour alternate-day fast is a reasonable goal while eating whole foods on feeding days (see Appendix A, week four). If 24 hours seems to be too long, you could start with as little as 12 hours per day, which is basically our sleeping time, working up to 16 to 18 hours a day and continuing to work up to 24 hours. So, on the 24-hour alternate-day fast, you would eat dinner one evening then not eat again until dinner the following night, only drinking

allowed fluids. Then the following day you would eat normally and then repeat the process.

There are times that you will have to switch from one fasting regimen to another. This is because occasionally you will hit plateaus in your progress. Remember, the body likes to resist weight loss as we have previously mentioned, so by changing up the regimen it changes the body's ability to hinder progress. For a more detailed look at other fasting options and time periods, I would refer you to *The Complete Guide to Fasting* by Dr. Fung.

Now, once you reach your therapeutic goal (desired weight, lowered sugar numbers, etc.), you will want to proceed to a maintenance program. This is where most people make a big mistake. They think that once they reach their goal, they are finished and return to their old ways of eating. This would begin the trek back to their original bad health. What is needed at this point is a plan that will keep you at your desired result permanently which, hopefully, becomes a new lifestyle.

There are many options for maintaining your new found health. It may take some experimentation to determine the most effective plan. One option would be to decrease fasting times to one or two 24-hour fast per week. You would continue to eat whole nutritious foods during feeding times. Another option would be to skip a meal once a day on an ongoing basis, preferably breakfast. That would give you an ongoing 16 - 18 hour intermittent fast. Again, the idea is for you to find the plan that keeps you at your desired therapeutic result. This maintenance program is what distinguishes this plan from any other diet program. It will continue to reset and reboot the mitochondria (the energy makers of each cell in the body). This is very important because this will maintain cellular vitality and integrity. If you can keep the mitochondria healthy your odds of maintaining good health greatly increase. Another benefit is that it keeps the insulin levels low which prevents it from creeping back up to a new "set" level. This will hold your weight and sugar at the desired levels.

Ooops. I just had to eat!
I would like to add one other note. Many people will give up on their intermittent fasting plan because they prematurely break the fast. This usually happens because they get hungry and just have to eat something or they're put into a situation in which they have to eat, such as a business lunch or some other function. It's okay. There is no condemnation. Just pick it up and start over and keep going. It's no big deal. This is a marathon, not a sprint. When you

start again, the insulin levels will lower and you'll be back on track.

What am I supposed to eat?

This can become a very complicated subject so I'm going to try to make it as simple as possible. CARBOHYDRATES equal sugar. Eat a bunch of carbs and your pancreas and liver will go into the "Bob" mode. You want to eat natural whole nutritious foods. This is pretty much accomplished when you eat foods high in fat and moderate protein and very low in carbohydrates. Don't do a Bob and drink fruit juices due to the amount of fructose (see the chapter on sugars). Anything with grains is going to be high in carbohydrates and therefore cause inflammation in the body. What makes matters worse are all grains in modern western civilization have been highly refined and go straight to blood sugar. Perhaps the only grain that can be eaten in very small quantities is rice. Here is a snapshot of what is low in carbs and will help you in your journey to longevity.

Meat/Protein: Eggs, Beef, Poultry, Seafood, Pork, Lamb

Low carb vegetables: (iceberg lettuce, celery, spinach, Brussel sprouts, kale, cauliflower, zucchini, asparagus, etc.)

Real Cheese: Gouda, Goat, Swiss, Cheddar, Cottage cheese sparingly.

Fats & Oils: Avocado, Coconut oil, Olives & Olive oil

Nuts and Seeds: Almond, walnuts, pecans, etc. Various nut butters, especially for snacks

Real Butter & Whole Cream: (No half and half), Ghee is also good.

Eating times have suddenly become simple. There is no diet plan to follow. There are no shakes, or bars, or smoothies. Eat as much as you want during meals. Just eat healthy. As long as you stay within your low carb food groups and fast you will lower insulin and lose weight. But, if you try to eat all of these fats and proteins combining them with high-carbs, well, if you're not as big as Bob now, you're going to be! That said, everyone has a weakness. Pizza is Bob's. He is trying to get his life on the straight and narrow, but he is not perfect. There was that late-night leftover pizza slice that didn't survive until morning. He ate it. He owned up to it. And went back on the wagon. Don't lose heart. If you fall down face first into a slice of red velvet cake, just pick yourself up and get back to fasting!

Intermittent Fasting is a lifestyle!
(not just another diet program)

1. **Start!**
   - Start intermittent fasting at whatever pace you feel comfortable with.
   - For example, you could start with fasting 12 hours every day. That's sleeping time.
2. **Keep it Simple!**
   - If you have to prematurely break the fast, just start over again.
3. **Stay Hydrated**
   - Stay well hydrated using sea salt, trace minerals and water containing lemon.
4. **Increase your fasting to build health and reach goals.**
   - Next move to a daily 16-18 hour fast. That's basically skipping breakfast. No snacks!
   - Work your way up to preferably a 24 hour-alternating day fasting schedule eating maybe 2 meals consisting of whole foods on feeding days.
5. **Include a new eating paradigm.**
   - To control insulin, you need to reduce or eliminate carbohydrates.
   - When you eat, think Paleo or Ketogenic.

- You should restrict fruits, and fruit juices if trying to lose weight.
- On fasting days, you can drink coffee with heavy whipping cream, water, teas, organic bone broth, and bulletproof coffee.

6. **Make plans to maintain your new health after reaching goals.**

- Once you have reached your therapeutic goal, a maintenance program should be started i.e. 24-hour fast 1 - 2 times per week or 16-18 hour fast every day.

Things to Remember:

Let's age well.
- ✓ Let's "reboot" our bodies to attain our goals of "aging well."
- ✓ Intermittent fasting is a key component to this reboot as it will:
  - ○ empty the cells of the body of old fats and sugars
  - ○ lower blood insulin levels which makes it easier to lose weight
  - ○ reset the mitochondria - the energy makers in each cell in our body.
- ✓ Bad eating habits of sugar, flour, and high carbohydrates are what got you into trouble to

begin with. Don't cheat! Whether it is Paleo or Ketogenic, stick to your new eating paradigm and don't "backslide."

Let's lose weight.
- ✓ We must deal with the insulin issue in order to lose weight.
- ✓ Fasting is more about changing your body's physiology and endocrinology (hormonal picture) back to its original design.
- ✓ Intermittent fasting allows the body to reset insulin to a lower level which allows the body to burn fat which results in losing weight.
- ✓ Body weight has to be reset to its "set" weight - intermittent fasting accomplishes this.

Let's feel better.
- ✓ Intermittent fasting allows the body to shift into a healing mode.
- ✓ Intermittent fasting reduces inflammation which decreases pain and improves digestion.
- ✓ When you eat, you're telling your body to store food energy. When you don't eat, insulin levels drop and you burn food energy.
- ✓ Plateaus could be congested organs that would need to be flushed.
- ✓ The lymphatic system must be open and flowing to eliminate toxins.

- ✓ Moderate exercise is encouraged - walking, swimming, light weight lifting.
- ✓ A regimen of nutrition must be maintained which would include **multiple vitamin, multiple minerals, oils, sea salt, and coenzyme Q10.**

Let's press on to health and longevity.
- ✓ Remember, we're all on a journey to somewhere. Our 30's, 40's, 50's are heading to the 80's, 90's and beyond - what kind of health will we be in when we get there.
- ✓ Intermittent fasting combined with eating good whole foods gives us a way to proactively take charge of our health.
- ✓ Don't give up.
  - ○ Give it thirty days, but know that it could take 6-8 weeks to begin to see results.
  - ○ Get a partner or a group to join you so you can encourage each other.
- ✓ And remember, you can do this.

So, as we conclude, I really believe that intermittent fasting and proper eating will not only change your physical health but will become transformational to your life. The mental and spiritual clarity I am personally experiencing is dramatic. Who would have thought that <u>not doing something</u> that is so natural to do, that is eating, would have such a dynamic effect on our lives?

We really should not be surprised. It was God who designed us, and gave us the Bible as a "manufacturer's operating manual." There in the midst of the pages of His manual we find the principle of regular, intermittent fasting.

APPENDIX A:

A sample one-month start-up protocol to help get you on your way. You have the option to jump in anywhere in the protocol depending on your desire and level of urgency. You may speed up or slow down the process to your liking. There's really no right or wrong in how you approach this. The purpose is to ease you into the fasting protocol.

Week One

Let's start very simply. Begin by removing one of your snacks per day. Begin to remove sugars and desserts. Start reducing sodas and other sugary drinks. If you're eating more than three meals per day, skip one of them.

Week Two

Eliminate all snacking, particularly after dinner. By eliminating after dinner snacking, you are entering a 12-hour fasting period between dinner and breakfast. The good news is that you'll be sleeping through most of this fast. Start removing high glycemic carbohydrates such as bread, pasta, white potatoes and grains. Start eating meats, vegetables, healthy fats and the foods listed in chapter 13.

Week Three

Eat two meals within an eight-hour window. Do this three days this week. Continue with eating whole foods when eating and drink the allowable drinks when fasting. You're now fasting 16 hours a day on fasting days.

Week Four

You're now going to start your 24-hour alternate day fasting. This is how it works:

Every other day you will eat at the meal time of your choosing (breakfast, lunch or dinner). Let's say you choose dinner. You'll not eat again until dinner the next day, drinking only the approved drinks. This will be on Monday, Wednesday, Friday. Then on Sunday, Tuesday, Thursday, Saturday, you will go back to eating within your eight-hour window above in week three. You should now be eating only low carb whole foods out of the Keto-Paleo world (See Appendix B) and drinking approved drinks.

APPENDIX B:

ACCEPTABLE NUTRITIONALLY DENSE FOODS FOR EATING DAYS

To simplify this food list, it has been divided into the three generalized categories of foods, CARBOHYDRATES, HEALTHY FATS, AND PROTEINS

A DRINK and SNACK list is also included:

NUTRIENT AND MINERAL RICH CARBOHYDRATES

VEGETABLES with * limit due to higher sugar content

Arugula
Artichokes
Asparagus
Bok choy
Broccoli
Brussel Sprouts
Butterhead Lettuce
Cabbage
*Carrots
Cauliflower
Celery
Chard
Chicory Greens
Chives
Cucumber
Dandelion Greens
Eggplant
Endives
Fennel
Garlic
Jicama
Kale
Kohlrabi
Leeks
Leafy Greens
Mustard Greens
Mushrooms
Okra
Olive
*Onions
Parsley
Assorted Peppers
Pickles
*Potato (assorted)
Pumpkin
Radish
Romaine Lettuce
Scallion
Seaweed
Shallots
*Spaghetti Squash
Spinach
Swiss Chard
*Tomatoes
Turnip Greens
Watercress
Zucchini
Sauerkraut

HERBS AND SPICES

Allspice
Basil
Cardamom
Cayenne Pepper
Chili Powder
Cinnamon
Cilantro
Cloves
Coriander
Cumin
Curry Powder
Dill
Ginger
Italian Seasoning *(No Sugar added)*
Oregano
Paprika
Rosemary
Thyme
Turmeric
Sage

FRUIT - *NO JUICE*

Avocado
Blackberry
Blueberry
Lemon
Lime
Raspberry
Strawberry

(OTHER)
Almond Flour
Cacao Nibs/Powder
Coconut Flour
Coconut Aminos
Coconut unsweetened
100% Dark Chocolate
Mustard
Tamari Sauce *(Gluten Free)*
Vanilla Extract
Vinegars

HEALTHY FATS
Avocados
Avocado Oil
Coconut Butter/Oil
Ghee *(Clarified Butter)*
MCT Oil
Olive Oil
Sesame Oil/Walnut Oil *(small amounts)*

NUTS AND SEEDS
Almonds
Cashews
Chia Seeds
Flaxseed
Hazelnuts
Macadamia Nuts
Peanuts *(limited)*
Pecans
Pine Nuts
Pumpkin Seeds
Sesame Seeds
Sunflower Seeds
Walnuts
Assorted Nut Butters
(Organic Peanut, Organic Cashew, Organic Almond etc.)

FULL FAT DAIRY – *choose Organic from grass fed animals when possible*
Blue Cheese
Organic butter
Organic Heavy Whipping Cream (NO HALF-HALF)
Organic Greek Yogurt (plain and unsweetened)
Organic cheeses from grass fed animals:
Brie
Cheddar
Cottage Cheese
Cream Cheese
Feta
Goat cheese
Gouda
Mozzarella
Ricotta Cheese
Swiss

PROTEINS
Eggs   Protein/fat

MEATS – *Choose from preferably Grass-Fed animals and prepared with no nitrates etc.*
Bacon
Beef
Bison
Chicken
(Game Meats – Turkey, Boar, Deer, Rabbit, Pheasant etc.)
Hot Dog *(All Beef/Turkey)*
Lamb
Luncheon meats
(Organ Meats – Bone Marrow, Heart, Kidney, Liver, Tongue, Tripe)
Pepperoni
Pork
Salami
Sausage

Turkey
Veal
Snacks: Beef Jerky, Pork Rinds

SEAFOOD
Anchovies
Bass
Clams
Cod
Crab
Flounder
Grouper
Haddock
Halibut
Herring
Lobster
Mackerel
Mahi Mahi
Orange Roughie
Perch
Red Snapper
Salmon
Sardines
Shrimp
Scallops
Sole
Squid
Tilapia
Trout
Tuna

DRINKS - (No Carrageenan - Additive)
Almond Milk
Broth (Beef, Bone, Chicken, Vegetable)
Cashew Milk
Club soda/Seltzer water/Sparkling Mineral Water
Coconut Milk

Coffee
Bulletproof coffee
Herbal Teas
Unsweet Teas
Spring Water – *(Add a splash of lemon or lime with a pinch of Sea Salt for an exceptional hydrating drink)*

SNACKS

½ Avocado
Beef Jerky
¼ cup Berries (Blackberries, Blueberries, Raspberries, or Strawberries)
1 oz. Cheese/Cheese stick
Celery sticks
Cucumber
Hard Boiled Egg/Deviled Egg
Cold meat (Leftovers, luncheon meats like Ham, Roast Beef, Salami, Chicken etc.)
1 Tbls. Nut Butter
¼ cup Almonds/Cashews/Pecans or/Walnuts
Pork Rinds
Small Dinner Salad
½ Can of Tuna

ABOUT THE AUTHOR

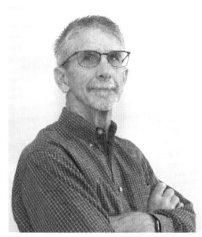 Dr. Grady Goolsby has been a chiropractic physician for over 41 years, with his primary focus being functional or nutritional medicine. His professional training was conducted at the National College of Chiropractic in Lombard, Illinois, where he received his Doctor of Chiropractic degree and received certifications in acupuncture and sports injuries. He did his internship in the inner city of Chicago, with the Chicago General Health Services.

Upon graduation, he returned to his home state of Florida and began private practice which focused primarily on musculoskeletal issues, sports injuries, and personal injury cases. However, he always longed to be involved in the world of nutrition, herbology, homeopathy, and energy medicine. In 1991, he began working in a medical facility that specialized in intravenous chelation therapy and metabolic medicine, which continued for seven years. In the meantime, he was introduced to Dr. D.A. Versendaal, the inventor and teacher of Contact Reflex Analysis, an analytical technique to determine nutritional deficiencies through the acupuncture meridian system. Dr. Versendaal became one of Dr. Goolsby's mentors and greatly influenced his training in functional nutritional medicine.

Today Dr. Goolsby continues his private practice in Florida. Along with chiropractic care, he provides patients with information on nutrition, evidenced-based whole food supplements, intermittent fasting, diet, chemical and heavy metal avoidance, and energy medicine to prevent disease and promote healthy lifestyles. Patients continue to seek his consultation from all over the world.